It was ready.

Hugo turned the barbecue down, piled all the food on the warming rack and closed the lid.

He turned, his mouth open to speak, and then stopped.

“Ellie?” His voice was low, no more than a murmur, but she didn’t respond, and his mouth softened into a rueful smile. He didn’t have the heart to wake her.

Her chest was rising and falling slowly, her limbs relaxed, and he made himself look away. He really didn’t need to know what she looked like when she was asleep, her face unguarded, her body motionless apart from the gentle lift of her breasts toward the sun with every slow breath...

God, he wanted her. He wanted her so much it hurt, but she deserved so much more than he could offer.

He closed his eyes, but he could still see her, see the soft curves, the peep of cleavage in the vee of her top.

Should he wake her? She clearly needed to sleep.

T0303207

Dear Reader,

I've never been a plotter, always a pantser, and this book is a classic example of my fingers taking over from my brain! I'm so glad they did, because it gave me something I could really get hold of to throw in the way of true love. And after I found that magic ingredient, the words flew.

Hugo and Ellie are very dear to me. I really, really wanted them to get their happy ending, but it's been a long time coming, so apologies to anyone who's been waiting patiently for my next book! I do hope you love them both as much as I do.

So here they are for you, with my love.

Caroline x

PS: Talking of magic ingredients, if you feel like trying out Sarah Rossi's Marry Me Chicken recipe, I found it on *Taming Twins*, and it's turned into a character all by itself!

A VET TO HEAL HIS HEART

CAROLINE ANDERSON

Harlequin

MEDICAL ROMANCE

If you purchased this book without a cover you should be aware that this book is stolen property. It was reported as "unsold and destroyed" to the publisher, and neither the author nor the publisher has received any payment for this "stripped book."

Harlequin® MEDICAL ROMANCE™

Recycling programs for this product may not exist in your area.

ISBN-13: 978-1-335-94274-6

A Vet to Heal His Heart

Copyright © 2024 by Caroline Anderson

All rights reserved. No part of this book may be used or reproduced in any manner whatsoever without written permission.

Without limiting the author's and publisher's exclusive rights, any unauthorized use of this publication to train generative artificial intelligence (AI) technologies is expressly prohibited.

This is a work of fiction. Names, characters, places and incidents are either the product of the author's imagination or are used fictitiously. Any resemblance to actual persons, living or dead, businesses, companies, events or locales is entirely coincidental.

For questions and comments about the quality of this book, please contact us at CustomerService@Harlequin.com.

TM and ® are trademarks of Harlequin Enterprises ULC.

Harlequin Enterprises ULC
22 Adelaide St. West, 41st Floor
Toronto, Ontario M5H 4E3, Canada
www.Harlequin.com

Printed in U.S.A.

Caroline Anderson is a matriarch, writer, armchair gardener, unofficial tearoom researcher and eater of lovely cakes. Not necessarily in that order! What Caroline loves: Her family. Her friends. Reading. Writing contemporary love stories. Hearing from readers. Walks by the sea with coffee/ice cream/cake thrown in! Torrential rain. Sunshine in spring/autumn. What Caroline hates: Losing her pets. Fighting with her family. Cold weather. Hot weather. Computers. Clothes shopping. Caroline's plans: Keep smiling and writing!

Books by Caroline Anderson

Harlequin Medical Romance

Yoxburgh Park Hospital

Best Friend to Wife and Mother?
Their Meant-to-Be Baby
The Midwife's Longed-For Baby
Bound by Their Babies
Their Own Little Miracle
A Single Dad to Heal Her Heart
From Heartache to Forever
Tempted by the Single Mom
The Midwife's Miracle Twins
Finding Their Forever Family

Healing Her Emergency Doc

Visit the Author Profile page
at Harlequin.com for more titles.

Huge thanks to Sarah Rossi at *Taming Twins* for the Marry Me Chicken recipe, the missing ingredient in the story without which this book would not be the same!

And, as ever, to my long-suffering and apparently endlessly patient editor, Sheila Hodgson, whose guiding hand has hauled me back from the brink on countless occasions over the past almost twenty-five years. Thank you from the bottom of my heart.

Praise for
Caroline Anderson

"What a delightful story.... Overall, Ms. Anderson has delivered an emotionally-animating and entertaining read in this book...the romance was nicely-detailed."
—*Harlequin Junkie* on *From Heartache to Forever*

CHAPTER ONE

FINALLY!

Ellie turned onto the drive with a sigh of relief and stared at her little house for a long moment.

She'd saved hard for a deposit and since she'd bought it three years ago as an investment she'd let it to tenants to cover the mortgage. She'd never lived in it herself because she hadn't needed to, but she did now, so thank goodness it was available.

It shouldn't have been. Wouldn't have been, if it hadn't been for her tenant doing a midnight flit a few weeks ago. She'd been furious at the time, but now she was grateful that it was empty, even if, in the words of the agent, it needed 'a little attention'. But that was fine. Thanks to Craig she had time on her hands now, if nothing else. Certainly no job security, that was gone and the rent-free flat that went with it…

No. She wasn't going down that rabbit hole again. Time to find out what 'a little attention' actually meant.

She sucked in a deep breath, then turned to look at Lola in the back seat. After six horrendous hours in heavy traffic, it wasn't just Ellie who was more than ready to get out of the car. Her little black Lab was sitting up now, her face expectant, tail wagging, and Ellie dredged up a smile.

'This is our new home, Lola. It's going to be great!'

Maybe her voice had been more convincing than she thought, or maybe the dog was just as relieved as she was, but she jumped up, and Ellie got stiffly out of the car, let her out and led her to the front door.

The paint was a little chipped and faded now, but that was hardly a major issue. She slipped her key in the lock, turned it and stepped inside.

And stopped.

A little attention? It smelt stale and unpleasant, and she wouldn't feel happy until she'd scrubbed it from top to bottom and cleaned all the carpets. Lola was busy sniffing, and she led her through the sitting room to the kitchen at the back and peered out of the window.

The light was fading, but she could see the once-tidy garden was a mess and heaven knows when the grass was last cut. Well, her agent had warned her, and it wouldn't take long to get it in order. Like the house, it was only tiny and easily manageable. She let Lola out for a wee and a sniff and left the door open while she went to check out the rest of the house.

She'd furnished it sparsely when she'd bought it three years ago, but everything was tired and dirty now, the mattress grubby, the bathroom filthy, and her optimism hit a brick wall. She came back down and sat with a plonk on the bottom step, her usually relentless optimism crushed.

What had she been thinking? Yes, she owned the house, but she knew nobody in Yoxburgh, and her rose-tinted family holidays here seemed worlds away. And the house was awful now. Beyond awful, really. 'A little attention' didn't even scratch the surface.

She sat up straight. No. She just needed to clean it, get the paintbrush out and—

The loud yelp made her turn her head sharply, and she ran out through the kitchen and found Lola limping towards the door. Even in the fading light she could see the thin spurt of blood from her right hind leg, and her heart went into overdrive.

'Lola! Oh, sweetheart…'

She needed a vet fast, but how to get her there before she bled out? She laid Lola down on her side, pressed her thumb firmly over the femoral artery high up in her groin above the wound to stop the bleeding, and studied it carefully. Whatever Lola had slashed herself on, she was pretty sure it wasn't glass. The cut wasn't clean enough for that, more a jagged tear, and it was just above her knee on the inside of her thigh, so she could get a pressure pad on it. If she had one…

She held her fingers on the artery while Lola whined and struggled to get free, stripping off her sweater and thin vest-top, swapping thumbs, then she balled the top up into as firm a wad as she could manage one-handed and wrapped her scarf tightly around it to hold it in place over the wound.

Lola did her best to resist, and at one point she put her teeth on Ellie's hand, not hard, just a gentle protest, but Ellie knew it must be very painful for her.

'Good girl, it's OK, I've got you, sweetheart, it's going to be all right,' she murmured, but she wasn't sure if it was. Tying it tight enough to stop the bleeding was next to impossible, and Lola wasn't helping, but it was as tight as she could get it and at least it had slowed the blood flow down.

So now what?

Back to the car and head to the nearest vet. She'd been scoping out the practices online this morning with the intention of visiting them to ask about locum work, and the closest by miles was just three streets away in a big old Victorian house. She'd driven past it on the way here, and they had excellent reviews. She tugged her sweater back on hurriedly, carried Lola to the car and set off, praying that the makeshift tourniquet would stay put until she'd got there.

Please be open, please be open, please be open...

There! Yoxburgh Veterinary Practice. She swung through the open gates into the empty car park in front of the building, jumped out and ran to the door. She could see lights on at the back, but the entrance was in darkness, and her heart sank. She rang the bell and pounded on the heavy old door.

Please be open...

Nothing. She fumbled for her phone and rang the practice, and was automatically transferred to the night service. It was miles away, but she'd been watching the wound as she'd phoned, and she could see the blood slowly seeping through the wadded-up top and her scarf every time she took her hand off the pad.

If she didn't get help soon, Lola was going to die.

She felt a sob rise in her throat as she hung up and pressed hard on the pad, and Lola whined and licked her hand.

'Oh, baby. I can't lose you, not like this, not now after everything else…'

She fought down the sobs, kneeling on the edge of the back seat and stroking her sweet, gentle dog with her other hand while she tried to work out what she could do. Move her to the front seat so she could reach to press on the pad as she drove? No, the front seat and footwell were packed to window height and it would take too long.

So—leave her in the back and drive fast? She couldn't, not that fast. If she took the pressure off she'd bleed out in minutes, and the tourniquet, such as it was, had already been on nearly ten minutes.

Five more minutes and the leg would be compromised…

Stay there all night pressing on it until the surgery opened again, and resign herself to Lola losing her leg?

Or just pray for a miracle?

So much for their new start. If only she'd stayed put—but she couldn't have, not after what had happened, and now everything was falling apart and Lola was going to die. She'd never felt so helpless in her life.

She went back to the door and pounded on it again.

'Where *are* you?' she wailed. 'Why won't you open the door?'

But they didn't. Whoever was in there was ignoring her, and she went back to Lola, leant on the pressure pad again and stroked her head gently with a hand that shook with grief and guilt and horror.

'I'm sorry, sweetheart. I'm so, so sorry…'

* * *

The pounding on the door seemed frantic, and Hugo hesitated another few seconds and gave in.

He went out through the staff entrance, Rufus at his heels, and saw a car in the car park, the back door hanging open. A woman was half in, half out of it, giving him a distractingly tempting view of a gently rounded bottom in snug jeans.

He ignored the inappropriate urge and was gearing up to explain that the practice was closed when he heard a wrenching sob that made his heart sink. So much for his quiet Friday evening walk with Rufus…

He peered in at her. 'Can I help you?'

She turned her head, her face streaked with blood and tears, a strand of dark hair clinging damply to her cheek. He didn't wait for a reply, just told Rufus to stay and ran round to the other side of the car and opened the door.

A dog, a black Labrador by the look of it, still alive but bloodied and whimpering, and the woman was leaning on some kind of makeshift bandage on her hind leg.

'What happened?'

'No idea. I let Lola out into the garden and heard a yelp and she was hosing blood—'

'OK, let's get her inside. I'm Hugo, by the way. And you are?'

'Ellie.' Her eyes held his and he could see hope in them. 'You're the vet?'

'Yes.'

Another wrenching sob made her whole body convulse, and he took over, lifting the injured dog into his arms and carrying her swiftly round to the side door. He opened it with his elbow and went inside, Rufus beside him, and he sent him to his bed and headed straight through to the prep room, putting the dog down on the table.

'It's OK, Lola, I've got you, sweetheart,' he said gently, and the dog licked his hand and gave a quiet whimper. A trembling, bloodied hand reached out and stroked the dog's head, and he leant on the makeshift pressure pad and looked up and met Ellie's distraught eyes.

'Right, tell me everything you know.'

Her voice had a tremor, but her words were calm and concise. 'It's her femoral artery. No idea what she tore it on, I'd just let her out for a wee, but it's a jagged cut, so most likely not glass. I did what I could to contain it, but she's probably lost two hundred mils, maybe more?'

He gave an inward eyeroll. She'd probably spent her life watching vet programmes. 'That's a wild guess,' he said, but she cut that off with her next words.

'It's an educated wild guess. I'm a vet.'

He met her eyes again. 'Seriously?'

She rolled her eyes, echoing his thoughts, which under normal circumstances he would have found funny, but this wasn't exactly normal. But if she really was a vet…

'Do I look as if I'm joking? My dog is bleeding out, and that pressure has been on for about twelve minutes now! Can you please just give her a GA and clamp the artery before she bleeds to death or you have to amputate her leg?' Her voice cracked on that, and he frowned.

'I'll call my nurse—'

'You don't need a nurse, Hugo, I'm a vet! I've got all my paperwork in the car, or you could call my old boss James Harkness, but we don't have time for that now. Please—before it's too late?'

His mouth opened, but then he clamped it shut and held her eyes.

Come on, come on...

'You know Jim?'

'Yes. He owned my old practice. I worked with him for eight years.'

Another pause, then, 'OK,' he said at last, and her shoulders sagged with relief. 'Right,' he went on, stepping up a gear. 'You hold this while I get everything ready, and once I've got her under I can clamp that artery and get a proper look at it. Meanwhile tell me a bit more about her, please.'

She watched him, heart pounding, itching to do it herself, hoping he'd do things the way she would, and while he prepped at lightning speed, she filled him in.

'She's got no pre-existing conditions that I know of, no contra-indications, she weighs twenty kg. I gave her a general anaesthetic to drain an abscess at the back of her mouth three and a half weeks ago, she was fine for that and it's healed well. She hasn't eaten since this morning, she had a drink about three hours ago.'

'Good.' He was moving briskly and efficiently, doing what she would have done. Warming a bag of Hartmann's in hot water because Lola would need the compound sodium lactate solution to replace her lost blood volume, pulling up the induction agent, checking the anaesthetic gas in the vaporiser, selecting an ET tube, and she began to think they might after all be able to save Lola and her leg.

He clipped the hair on the front leg that hadn't been recently cannulated, asked her to hold it while he slid the needle in, and moments later Lola was asleep, intubated and out of pain. 'OK, let's move her into Theatre,' he said, and they carried her through and he connected her up to the gas. He was setting up fluids, injecting pain relief and antibiotics, checking Lola's stats, moving reassuringly swiftly. Then he looked up and met her eyes again.

'Right, we're good to go,' he said, then added, 'Which end do you want?' which surprised her.

The leg, because she wanted to know exactly what was going on in there, but she didn't know where anything was in his theatre, and anyway, her hands were shaking too much and vascular surgery needed steady hands. And she realised she trusted him.

Not that she had a choice…

'You do the leg, I'll monitor her.'

To her relief, he did exactly what she would have done.

Keeping his thumb on the artery, he removed the makeshift pressure pad, then released the pressure carefully.

Blood welled in the wound, but at least it didn't spurt.

'It might have closed up a bit,' she said hopefully, but as soon as she said that it started again, a thin stream streaking out across the room, and he shook his head and clamped the artery.

'OK, let's clean this up and get a better look. Up the fluids, please. We need to boost her circulation now.'

She'd already done it as soon as the artery forceps were on, and she watched as he filled the wound with sterile gel to protect it from the clipped hair, ran the clippers over the inside of Lola's thigh, scrubbed the skin with chlorhexidine, sucked out the gel and irrigated the wound thoroughly.

Just what she would have done. She heaved an inward sigh of relief.

'How's she doing?' he asked without looking up.

'She's fine. All good.'

He nodded, laid out all the instruments he'd need, then while he scrubbed she opened the outer packets ready for him.

'OK, let's get a good look at this.'

He laid a sterile drape over the leg, blotted the wound with a swab, and she leaned over and studied it with him. The artery was punctured, but it was also grazed, not extensively but enough that it would need a skilled vascular surgeon to fix it.

'That's a nasty graze. Can you repair it?' she asked without any real hope, but he shook his head.

'No. If it was just the tiny hole, I'd give it a go, but the graze has damaged the vessel wall and I don't have the equipment or skills for fine vascular surgery. It needs a graft.'

'So what do we do?'

'Tie it off and hope? The artery's been clamped for a few minutes but her foot's still warm, she has good perfusion of the tissues, so I reckon she's got a good enough supply from the other vessels. She should be fine, but realistically, we have no other options.' He looked up and met her eyes. 'Unless you want her to go to a specialist? We can probably get her stable enough. Up to you.'

She shook her head. 'No. I've tied it off in a similar case, and frankly, if she's got enough of a blood supply to that leg for it to survive the journey, it's probably fine anyway.'

He nodded, and his gloved fingers explored the wound carefully.

'Nothing in there that I can feel. You've got no idea at all what she cut it on?'

'No, none. I'd literally just got the keys off the rental agent and walked in, and I'd got no idea what's in the garden, so I should have been more careful.'

He raised an eyebrow. 'X-ray?'

She nodded. 'Might be an idea, as I haven't got a clue what it was. She was probably racing round like a mad thing. She'd been in the car for six hours.'

He winced, and she pulled a face.

'Yeah. Long story. I'll tell you later.'

He wondered what the story was, but it would keep.

He X-rayed the leg, studied the images closely and tried not to think about the scent of something delicate and delicious drifting from her hair as she leant close to look at the screen.

'I can't see anything,' she said.

'No, nor can I.' He straightened up and told himself to focus. 'OK, let's close it.'

He tidied up the wound, debriding the edges so they'd come together in a clean line, tied off the artery and then hesitated.

'Does it need a drain in the dead space so she doesn't get a seroma?' she asked, echoing his thoughts, and he nodded.

'I'd rather put it in and take it out if it's not needed than have to do it later. Negative pressure drain?'

'I would.'

He made a tiny hole through the skin to the centre of the wound, slid in the fine flexible tube and taped the drain in place, then repaired the muscle damage before he drew the edges of the wound together and closed it with a continuous soluble suture. Then he squeezed the empty drain bottle and attached it to create suction in the wound and watched as a thin trickle of pink-tinted serum filled the fine tube. He gave a satisfied nod and looked up. 'How's she doing?'

'Fine. Stable.'

'Good. I'll get some local into that so it's not too sore when she wakes up, and then let's bring her round and see how she is.'

He stepped away from the table, pulled off his gloves and gown and binned them while she monitored Lola.

She was slowly coming to, but still sleeping, her breathing slow but steady, and together they put her into a mesh vest, tucked the suction bottle into it up against her tummy and then Hugo carefully moved her into a kennel and covered her with a warm blanket.

Ellie sat down onto the floor beside the kennel, her legs suddenly too weak to hold her. Lola was alive, her foot was warm, and she wasn't going to die. She realised she was shaking uncontrollably, and she felt a gentle hand on her shoulder.

'Hey, it's OK. She's going to be all right.'

Hugo hunkered down beside her, his hand still on her shoulder, warm and reassuring, and she turned her head and met his eyes. They were the kindest eyes she'd ever seen, and she couldn't hold that gentle, understanding gaze. She turned her head away again and blinked back tears.

'Have you had anything to eat or drink recently?'

Recently? Hardly. She shook her head. 'Not since this morning. I had a bit of water when I stopped to let Lola out, but—no, not really.'

'I'll knock something up. You OK with pasta and pesto?'

'Um—yes, fine. Sounds lovely. Thank you.'

'Good. I might even have some parmesan.'

She dredged up a smile, suddenly realising how hungry she was. 'Even better.'

He went through a door into what she assumed was a staff room. She could hear him talking to his dog, the sound of a food bowl being chased around the floor, and he came back a couple of minutes later with a large mug full of steaming tea.

'It's got sugar in it—and don't argue, just drink it,' he said over his shoulder as he walked away again.

She didn't argue. She was beyond arguing, and his kindness suddenly overwhelmed her. She put the tea down, buried her face in her hands and gave in to the tears.

She was crying. He could hear her as he ran back downstairs from his flat with the ingredients from his fridge, the quiet sobs tugging at his overused heartstrings.

He wondered again what the 'long story' was. Something that had taken her alone on a six-hour journey, ending up in a rental place with a garden that was clearly unsuitable for a young, energetic dog like Lola. Or any dog, really, by the sound of it.

He dumped the fresh pasta into boiling water, drained it, stirred a hefty dollop of pesto into it, grated the parmesan generously over their brimming bowls and carried them through.

'Here you go,' he said, and sat down cross-legged beside her.

She'd stopped crying now, and he could see why. Rufus was curled up in her lap, and she was stroking him with one hand and nursing her mug with the other. He called the dog over to his side, and he lay down between them, sharing the love. She got the head end, he noted wryly.

He handed her a bowl, and she put the tea down and took it with a smile and a hand that was still shaking. Low blood sugar? Shock? Exhaustion?

All of the above, probably.

They ate in silence.

She was glad of that. She was too tired, stressed and hungry to engage in polite conversation, and it seemed he was, too.

But then it was done, her bowl scraped clean, and she put it down and met his eyes. They were slate blue, and she thought they could see to the bottom of her soul, but that kindness was still there in them and she felt oddly safe. 'Thank you. That was amazing. I really needed it.'

'Yeah, me, too.' He smiled, his mouth tipping up a little on one side. 'You'll feel better soon.'

'I do already,' she told him honestly. 'I can't believe how kind you've been. It's restored my faith in human nature.'

'I haven't billed you yet,' he reminded her with a wry smile, and she gave a fractured little laugh.

'No, you haven't, but I'm sure you will.'

He chuckled, then held out his hand. 'It's probably time we introduced ourselves properly,' he said. 'I'm Hugo Alexander, and this is my practice.'

She knew that already from her research last

night, but she took his hand—the warm, strong and yet gentle hand that had squeezed her shoulder and reduced her to tears, that had saved Lola's life and leg with quiet competence—and she smiled at him.

'Eleanor Radcliffe. Ellie to my friends,' she added, and he cocked his head on one side, a smile playing around his lips.

'So, *Ellie*,' he said with quiet emphasis, 'this long story…'

She looked away from those kind yet piercing eyes that would see too much and gave a little shrug. 'Oh. That. I'm sure you've heard it before. I was working in Jim's practice in the Cotswolds. He was a brilliant boss, but he was getting on and he wanted to retire, so he stepped back and made me senior vet, which was great for a while, but things had moved on, some of the equipment needed upgrading, and he didn't want to invest any more in it, so he decided to sell it to a corporate.'

'Was that a problem?'

'Not initially. The building needed investment, and it was going to get it, which had to be a good thing. And then within a year the corporate sent in a new senior vet over me.'

'Ah…'

She threw him a wry smile. 'It's not what you think. He was an ex from uni days. We'd had a brief relationship, I'd dumped him when I realised he was a lying, cheating snake, then he'd said stuff about me that wasn't true that caused a rift with my best friend—and then he reappeared in my life and got his revenge.'

'How?'

'Oh, picking fault here and there, snide remarks, trying to undermine me with my colleagues—it went on for months, then we had a row over Lola, and I lost it.'

He frowned. 'What kind of a row?'

She sighed and looked over her shoulder at Lola. 'Her owner brought her in. She'd been off her food for a day or so, could barely open her mouth and her eye was being pushed out of the socket by something—a tumour, an abscess—I didn't know and I couldn't see without an anaesthetic, but her owner said she couldn't afford it, didn't have insurance because it was too expensive—she was heartbroken.

'She loved Lola to bits but she wasn't well herself, she was struggling to look after her properly, and she was utterly distraught. She'd tried every rescue place she could find without success, and now, with this issue, she thought it would be better for Lola if she was dead than facing an uncertain future, so she asked me to put her to sleep. And she's three. There was nothing wrong with her apart from whatever was going on in her mouth, she's a beautiful dog and she didn't deserve to die. I couldn't let that happen.'

'So you treated her for nothing?'

She shook her head. 'No, because that wouldn't have solved the problem going forward, but I said I'd take her on, keep her myself, give her a home for life and she signed her over to me on the spot. It turned out to be a massive abscess at the back of her jaw. She'd yelped when she'd been chewing a stick in the woods a few days before, her owner had said, so it was probably blackthorn or hawthorn, but I drained the abscess and flushed it, it healed up really quickly, and I paid the bill.'

'So what was his problem?'

She sucked in a breath. 'I'd used my staff discount for her treatment, and then Craig refused to give it to me, billed me in full for the initial consult, the op, the drugs, the dispensing fee, the kennel time, the overnight care, even though I'd done all that myself while I was off duty… He said it was company policy, which was a crock of nonsense. A staff discount was in my contract and he knew it, but he said the dog hadn't been mine at the time of the first consultation, so technically it was down to the previous owner, and if I didn't pay up he'd bill her.'

He frowned. 'That's horrendous. So what did you do?'

'I paid it, because I didn't want her being hassled and I don't want a bad credit rating, so I told him exactly what I thought of him, finished my shift, wrote a stinking letter to the company, went up to my flat over the practice, packed up all my stuff, put it in the car and drove away with Lola. I spent last night in a dog-friendly motel, got up this morning, spoke to the rental agent and drove here.'

His eyes widened. 'So this was only yesterday? You were lucky to find a house to rent so quickly.'

'Oh, no, I didn't, it's mine. I've been letting it, but a few weeks ago the tenant did a flit and left it in a bit of a state, so I thought—well, I don't know what I thought, really, but maybe I'd been naïve imagining I could just drive up here and move in, but I can't live in it, not like it is. Maybe I should have been less impulsive and stayed, but I just—I couldn't even look at Craig any more I was so angry.'

'I can see that. So when was her op?'

'Three and a half weeks ago. The Monday.'

'And he's only just now decided to bill you?'

'Yes. He didn't know anything about it. He started a three-week holiday the day Lola came in, so he didn't know. Then someone said something about Lola, and he looked at the accounts yesterday afternoon, and it all hit the fan.'

Hugo leant back against the wall, taking it all in.

'Wow. That's quite a twenty-four hours you've had.'

She laughed, but it ended on a tiny sob. 'Tell me about it. And now my poor little house turns out to be lethal, filthy and—I can't take her back there, not with a wound, and I have nowhere else to go.'

'No family?'

'No, my mother's in Spain.'

No mention of a father. He wondered why. 'No boyfriend, partner, significant other?' he asked, realising as he'd said it that he was blatantly fishing.

'No other at all. Just me and Lola.'

She shot him a smile, but it didn't look convincing. 'So there you are. I'm jobless and unemployable, I have a broken dog, and my house is bordering on uninhabitable.'

He frowned again. 'Why?'

She stared at him. 'I just told you why. The tenant—'

'No, I mean why are you unemployable?'

'Are you serious?' She gave a tiny huff of laughter without a trace of humour. 'You didn't see my letter! And I'm in breach of contract because I didn't give three months' notice, so who's going to employ me with a record like that? And I didn't hold back when I talked to him, so I wouldn't fancy his reference,' she added with a wry smile.

He grunted. 'Yeah, I can imagine.' He studied her face. It was still streaked with blood, her sweater was on inside out, her tired green eyes were red-rimmed and exhausted, but she still had fight in her. Impressive.

He took a deep breath, let it out again, and said, 'I have an idea. Feel free to say no, if you want to, but I'm short-staffed tomorrow.' He rolled his eyes. 'That's nothing new, I'm permanently short-staffed, but the locum who was doing tomorrow morning is sick. If you can show me all the appropriate certification, how do you fancy covering the shift?'

'But what about Lola?' she asked without missing a beat, and he smiled. He wasn't in the slightest bit surprised that the dog was her first thought.

'Lola needs to stay in overnight, probably for at least two nights, and we have a bed in the office that the night vets used before the staffing situation got ridiculous. You're welcome to stay and look after her tonight, do the shift tomorrow, and when that finishes we can go over to your house and blitz it together.'

She stared at him. 'You'd do all that for me? For a perfect stranger you know nothing about?'

Her eyes were welling with tears, and he had to stifle the urge to wrap his arms around her and kiss the tears away. He gave himself a mental kick and stuck to the facts.

'I know quite a lot about you. I know you're a competent vet, I know your dog comes first, I know you did exactly what I would have done under the circumstances, and I'm not being entirely altruistic. I do need a vet for tomorrow. I need another vet, full stop, so you could look on it as an interview, if you like?'

'An *interview*?'

'That's what I said.'

She looked away, then looked back at him, her face awash with a whole raft of conflicting emotions, and he held his breath.

Ellie, please say yes...

CHAPTER TWO

ELLIE STARED AT HIM, trying and failing to read his expression.

Could it really be so simple?

She blinked away the tears and felt one slide down her cheek. She swiped it away crossly with her hand, and it came away tinged with blood.

She tried to laugh, but it cracked in the middle. 'Gosh, I'm such a mess. How can you even consider employing me?'

'How?' he asked, sounding incredulous. 'Because I need a vet? Because you clearly know what you're doing, and you're passionate about your job?'

'How on earth do you know that?'

'Because you took Lola on and treated her because it was the right thing to do, and today you stood your ground and made me help you. So that's twice she would have died if you hadn't stepped in to help her. You saved her life today under really tricky conditions—'

'No. *You* saved her life.'

'No. You did, by getting that tourniquet on, getting her here and making damn sure I helped you fix her.'

She felt her cheeks colour. 'Sorry, I'm not normally that pushy.'

'It's fine, you were fighting for Lola, and if it helps, I would have done exactly the same thing.'

She stared down at herself and laughed in despair. 'Look at me! My sweater's on inside out! How on earth did I do that?'

His mouth twitched, and he gave a soft chuckle that resonated inside her in a weirdly unsettling way.

'Er—one-handed, while you wrestled with a dog that I'm guessing wasn't being too cooperative? It's not rocket science and I imagine you had bigger things to think about.'

A vivid image of Lola struggling as she tied the scarf around her leg flashed into her mind, and she shuddered.

'I guess I did.'

Behind her, Lola gave a little whine, and she reached out and laid a hand on her head, stroking it gently. 'It's all right, Lola. I'm still here. It's OK, there's a good girl.'

Her tail thumped gently, and a wet tongue came out and licked Ellie's hand. She struggled up onto her elbows and looked around, clocking Hugo, and her tail thumped again.

'What a sweetheart,' he murmured, shifting

in beside Ellie, so close that she felt the breath jam in her throat as he held out his hand for Lola to sniff.

She licked it, then looked round at her leg.

'Leave it, Lola,' he said, easing her head back down gently and stroking her to distract her, and she sighed and settled again.

Then he sat back on his heels, and Ellie breathed again.

'She's going to need the cone of shame,' she said, trying to focus on Lola and not the lingering masculine scent of his body, and he nodded ruefully.

'Yes, she is, otherwise she'll have that drain out in a minute.' He cocked his head on one side. 'So—what's your answer?'

She turned her head and looked at him, just inches away, and the breath jammed in her throat again. Those slate-dark eyes, so kind, so mesmerising, so intense…

'Did you mean it?'

'What, that I need a vet? Absolutely.'

She laughed softly. 'No, I believe that. I meant about helping me clean the house.'

He frowned. 'Of course I meant it. Lola needs to rest, anyway, and the first thing we need to do is find out what she cut herself on and deal with it. So—locum tomorrow?'

'On one condition. I do the shift for free in exchange for your help.'

'That's ridiculous.'

'You haven't seen the house yet,' she pointed out, and then added, 'I don't want your charity, Hugo. Take it or leave it.'

She held her breath, and then he gave a soft huff of laughter that echoed through her again as he gave in.

'OK, I'll take it—but only if you do the shift in exchange for Lola's treatment.'

'What? No! Absolutely not.' Ellie shook her head firmly. 'Anyway there's no need. She's insured.'

That expressive eyebrow quirked at her. 'Is she? Even though you've had her less than a month?'

She had. Damn. 'I can pay you,' she said, wondering exactly how she was going to do that, but his mouth twitched, drawing her attention again to those firm, sculpted and oh-so expressive lips.

'Lord, you are stubborn.'

'I am,' she retorted, dragging her eyes and her mind off his mouth. 'So what's it to be?'

He let the smile out then, and her heart quickened. 'I'll take it.'

She smiled back, relief flooding her, her pride restored. 'Good. My paperwork's all buried in the car somewhere but I could call Jim?'

His smile was warm and it made her heart hitch. 'Yeah, do that. I did a practice rotation with him when I was training. He's a great guy. Be good to talk to him again.'

She pulled her phone out of her back pocket, glanced at the time to see if it was too late and decided that nine fifteen would be OK. She rang him, and he answered immediately.

'Jim, it's Ellie. I have an odd request. I'm with Hugo Alexander, and—'

'Hugo? Really? How is he?'

She laughed. 'Stressed and overworked, I think. He's looking for a locum. Could you vouch for me, please?'

'Of course I can. Put him on.'

She handed the phone over, and watched Hugo's face as Jim spoke. At length. Hugo looked across at her, his eyes alight, that expressive mouth twitching. 'So you rate her, then, Jim?' he asked, and Jim started again.

'I'll take that as a yes. Thank you.' He was silent for a moment, then added, 'Ah. You'd better ask her that,' and he handed the phone back. 'He wants to know how come you're here.'

Jim's voice was concerned. 'Ellie? What's happened?'

'Yeah, I had a bit of an issue with the new senior vet. We have previously, and I—er—I walked out. Long story, I'll tell you another time, but it's not your fault. This was strictly personal and a bit of a vendetta on his part.'

'Oh, Ellie, I'm so sorry,' Jim said heavily.

'Don't be. It's not your fault, Jim, you did what was right for you and right for the practice. You had no control over who they hired, and neither did I.'

'No, apparently not, but it sounds like you're well out of it. You'll be all right with Hugo, though. He's a good lad. You can trust him.'

She hoped so, because right then she was all out of options. She said goodbye, hung up, met his eyes and raised a brow. 'Well?'

'According to Jim, you're the best vet he's ever had. I reckon that'll do me.'

He unfolded his legs and stood up, picked up their empty bowls and held out a hand, pulling her to her feet and sending tingles all the way down her arm.

'Why don't you get some fresh clothes from your car and see if you can find that paperwork, and I'll get the buster collar for Lola and keep an eye on her. There's a shower out the back, I'll find you a towel. And leave your clothes outside the shower, I'll throw them in the washing machine to get the blood off.'

She emerged from the shower feeling infinitely more civilised, to find he'd taken her clothes away. He'd also changed, so she guessed his scrubs were in the wash, too. And he'd put a pile of bedding in the office for her.

'I thought you might want to sleep next to Lola. You know, so you can hear the second she moves?'

She felt her shoulders drop as yet another worry fell away from her. 'That would be amazing. I was contemplating setting an alarm to check on her every half hour.'

He frowned. 'You can't do that. You need your sleep. You've got another long day tomorrow. I've topped up her pain relief, but she'll need to go out before you go to bed.'

She nodded. 'Where can I take her?'

'I'll show you, I've got to take Rufus out anyway now. I normally set the burglar alarm when I knock off, but I'll show you how it works so you can set it and unset it in the night if you need to take her out again.'

He led her out through the kitchen at the back, and into a garden. She wasn't expecting that, somehow, but as the light came on automatically she could see a large square of lawn with shrubs and trees around the sides against the old red brick walls, and an area of paving with some seating.

Rufus trotted off and started sniffing around, and Lola followed, limping a little unsteadily down the gentle ramp, then making her way onto the grass. She didn't bother to sniff, just bopped down awkwardly.

'Good girl,' Ellie said softly when she was done, and the dog turned and made her way back inside to her kennel without a fuss, lying down and letting out a big sigh.

'She's doing well.'

'She is. I'm so grateful to you—'

He rolled his eyes. 'You're like a stuck record. Wait till tomorrow, I'll get my own back.'

She somehow didn't think so. Nothing she did could ever make up for his care and kindness, but doing that shift for him might go some small way to redress the balance.

'I found my paperwork,' she told him. 'It's on the desk in the office.'

'Great. I'll take a look in the morning. Right, let's get this cone on Lola so she can't rip the drain out while you're asleep, and then I'll move your bed.'

They had to shoo Rufus off the folding bed before they moved it out beside Lola's kennel, and he showed her where the light switches were, put on a dim nightlight so she could see Lola, and showed her how to set and unset the alarm, a necessary evil because the drugs on the premises were a prime target.

Then he handed her a slip of paper. 'My mobile number. Call me if you're worried about her and I'll come down. I live over the practice.'

That didn't surprise her, she'd done it herself until last night, and lots of vets with small practices did the same. It was the 'I', not 'we', that struck her, but it might not be significant. And anyway, it was none of her business.

'Thank you. I'm sure she'll be fine. Will my

car be OK outside? It's just it's got my whole life in it right now.'

'It should be if you've locked it. I'm about to close the gates and there's CCTV on the drive.'

She felt another layer of stress peel away and smiled at him. 'That's great. Thank you.'

He went out through the side door and she watched him go, her mind whirling as she made up the bed.

He needed a vet. He wanted her to 'interview' for the post by doing the shift tomorrow. Was he serious? And would she contemplate it, so soon after the fall-out of the last one? But Jim had called him a 'good lad' and said she could trust him, and he'd been nothing but kindness…

He came back in then, cutting off her tumbling thoughts.

'Right, that's me done. Help yourself to anything you want in the kitchen, and shout if you need me. I'll be down here by seven. Sleep tight.'

Not a chance. She had far too much to think about. She dredged up a tired smile. 'You, too. And thank you, Hugo. For everything.'

His eyes creased into an answering smile that did something strange to her midsection. 'You're welcome. Rufus, come on, you're not sleeping there,' he said, and Rufus hopped down off her bed and trotted after him.

They went through a doorway, and she heard

his footsteps recede as they made their way up, leaving her alone with Lola and her thoughts.

Did she want to work here? Maybe—and maybe not, or not long term. But—locum? At least that way she'd have an income while she decided.

She lay down fully dressed, with her head close to Lola's kennel so she could see her just by turning her head. She'd settled down, and after a moment Ellie heard a gentle snore.

Poor Lola. What a start to their new life together, but at least they wouldn't starve, so maybe it wasn't going to be so bad after all…

She slept surprisingly well, and so, to her relief, did Lola.

She picked up her phone and looked at the time.

Six forty-three. He'd said he'd be down by seven, so she threw off the covers and got up, turned off the burglar alarm and checked on Lola.

She wagged her tail but didn't move. Not surprising, really. Her leg would be sore this morning, now the pain relief had worn off, but she hadn't complained once in the night and she'd accepted the cone without argument.

She put the fold-up bed away in the office, coaxed Lola out of her kennel, took her out for a sniff and a wee, then put her back in her kennel, had a quick wash and was heading for the kitchen when she heard the light patter of little feet running down the stairs, followed by a heavier tread, and Hugo and Rufus came through the door.

'Morning,' he said cheerfully, all freshly showered and smelling delicious. He handed her a neatly folded pile of yesterday's clothes.

'Gosh, that was quick! Thank you.'

'Pleasure. How are you both today? Did you sleep?'

'Better than expected,' she said with a wry laugh, trying not to think about how good he smelt. 'That bed is seriously comfy and Lola slept all night.'

'Good. I'll have a look in a minute. Ready for the fray?'

'I will be when I've eaten something. Can I make some toast?'

'Sure. Stick a couple of bits in for me while I have a look at Lola. Has she been out?'

'Yes. She seems fine, but a bit sore, I think.'

'I'm sure. I'll give her another shot. I just want to check her leg for the circulation, make sure it's not cold or swelling—'

'It isn't. It feels fine, which is a relief. I just wish I knew what she'd cut it on.'

'Well, we'll find out later, won't we? How about the drain?'

'The bottle had a little in. I left it for you to see.'

'Have you fed her?'

'No, not yet. Her food's somewhere in the car, but it's buried. I'll get it.'

'Is she a fussy eater?'

She laughed. 'She's a Labrador. What do you think?'

His mouth twitched. 'I'll give her something bland, then, see how she gets on with it. She may not want much.'

'Tea or coffee?'

'Coffee. White, no sugar. There's a machine in the corner and pods on the side.'

To his relief, Lola's foot was warm and not swollen and the drain was doing its job. She greeted him with a wag of her tail and a lick, and didn't even flinch when he gave her the painkilling injection, just inhaled her breakfast and lay down again. She was very lame, but that was to be expected, and she'd accepted the plastic cone around her head without too much fuss.

She seemed an utter sweetheart, and he could absolutely see why Ellie had refused to put her to sleep. He would have done the same under the circumstances. *Had* done the same, hence Rufus, and he hadn't regretted it for a moment.

He sorted out the suction drain, then went back to the kitchen, drawn by the smell of toast and coffee. They took it through to the office and after he'd looked through her paperwork they went through the morning's appointments together.

'OK, I've switched things around a bit, given you all the routine stuff, but we've got Kerry in, she's our head nurse, and she'll be able to give you a hand if you can't find anything. Oh, and I've found you some scrubs to wear.'

He showed her how the computer system worked, then swivelled round and met her eyes. 'Any questions?'

Too many.

She was still reeling with the shock of the last forty-eight hours, and she was glad he'd given her the simple consults, but there would still be much she didn't know about the practice.

'Can you give me a quick guided tour?'

'Sure.'

He got up and led her through a door to the reception desk in a corner of the waiting room. It was a lovely room, with a bay window to the front, high ceilings and ornate plaster cornicing. There was a screened waiting area for cats, and across the hall, past the lobby with the beautiful old front door she'd pounded on last night, was the main waiting room and doors to the two consulting rooms. They had doors at the back leading via a corridor to the stock room and pharmacy, the X-ray room and the areas she'd already seen. These areas, unlike the waiting rooms and entrance at the front, were modern, crisp and clinical. Pretty standard fare, really, and nothing she hadn't seen before, but spotlessly clean and very well equipped.

'Happy?'

She nodded, feeling a flicker of nerves, the word 'interview' hovering in the back of her mind. Actually, make that front…

'I'm fine.'

Her list of consults had been, as he'd promised, simple and straightforward, and Kerry had been a huge help. She'd also kept an eye on Lola, and said she was doing fine.

One less thing to worry about.

She saw her last client of the morning and was just filling in the details on the computer when there was a tap on the door and Hugo stuck his head round.

'Are you done?'

'Pretty much. I'm just writing the last one up.'

He closed the door and propped himself against it, somehow sucking all the air out of the room. 'How did you get on? Was everything OK?'

Was it? She'd thought so, but maybe Kerry had raised some concerns?

'I think so.'

'Kerry thinks so, too. She basically told me if I don't offer you the job she's going to walk.' He shrugged away from the door and shot her a grin that turned her heart inside out. 'Fancy a quick sandwich before we go and tackle the house?'

'Um—yes, please, that would be great. I'll just finish up here.'

He nodded and walked out, and she stared after him.

Had he just offered her a job?

Maybe… And maybe she was reading too much into it. She closed the file, shut down the computer and followed him out.

While Ellie took Lola out to the garden for a moment, he loaded his car with milk, teabags and a packet of biscuits, the carpet shampooer and cleaning stuff and some gardening tools, then once Lola was settled he put Rufus in his crate in the office and followed Ellie to her house.

It was small, modern, unprepossessing but innocuous—until you got inside.

'Hmm,' he grunted, and Ellie looked over her shoulder and gave him a wonky little smile.

'See what I mean?'

His answering smile felt every bit as crooked. 'Well, you didn't lie, let's put it like that.'

He followed her through the tired and grubby living room into the kitchen. 'This looks OK. I think you can rescue it with a bit of elbow grease.'

'I can, it just needs a good scrub. The rest is harder—especially the garden.'

He nodded, a glance through the window

enough to make his heart sink. Then she opened the back door, and the full story of last night's horror with Lola was revealed.

'Wow,' he murmured, staring at the stains all over the paving. 'She really was hosing blood.'

'She was. It's a miracle I managed to slow it enough to get her to you. Goodness knows what's lurking in the grass to tear her to shreds.'

Whatever it was, he couldn't see it. It was well and truly hidden by the overgrown grass and the tangle of weeds. No wonder she'd felt so defeated last night. Time to sort it out.

'Right,' he said briskly, 'I'll find out what tried to kill her in the garden while you tackle the kitchen, then we can have a cup of tea and work out a plan for the rest of the house.'

Ten minutes later she was on her knees scrubbing the kitchen floor when he propped himself up in the open doorway.

'I think I've found the culprit. There's a coil of barbed wire with a loose end hanging out into the grass, and there's blood and hair on one of the barbs. I'm guessing that's what she caught her leg on. Come and see.'

She followed him out and studied the wire thoughtfully. 'I think you're right. It's the right height, and it looks vicious enough. Poor Lola.'

He shot her a sympathetic smile. 'Absolutely.

And poor you, too. Did you say you had a letting agent?'

She suppressed a sigh. 'Yes.'

'Well, I have to say I don't think they earned their commission, not by the look of it. I would have thought at the least they'd have had it cleaned up.'

'I told them not to bother. He said it needed a little attention, so I'd already booked a week's leave to come up here to clean it. I just ended up coming a day early, but I think he might have been a tad frugal with the truth.'

The snort said it all, and she smiled wryly. 'Yeah. My thoughts entirely. Shall we drag the wire out of the grass so you can mow it and find out what else lurks beneath?'

'I've got a better idea. You go back in and finish cleaning up the kitchen, and I'll sort this out.'

It wasn't just the barbed wire—not that that wasn't bad enough, but he ended up going over the mercifully small lawn with a fine-tooth comb and pulling out all sorts of stuff that had just been dumped. Plastic bottles, nappies, broken crockery, a bamboo cane from some long-dead house plant, the occasional brick…

And until it was all out, he couldn't cut the grass.

He tipped the last lot of rubbish into the bin and headed for the kitchen door, just as she opened it.

'I've made some tea. Are you finished?'

He laughed at that. 'Not exactly. I've got the worst of it, so I might run the strimmer over it next and then rake it all off.'

'After you drink tea and have a biscuit,' she said, handing him a mug. 'Sorry about the chip, the crockery seems to have suffered along the way.'

'Yeah, I found some in the grass, along with everything else.'

'I'm not surprised. Come in and sit down. You should be safe, I washed the chairs.'

Two hours later they were back at the practice, tired but satisfied with their progress. The kitchen was clean, the sitting room was almost respectable, and she felt much more positive.

And grateful, because Hugo had been a Trojan in the garden, and it looked worlds better—which was just as well, as Lola was going to have to start using it very soon.

Immediately, if it hadn't been for Hugo's insistence that Lola couldn't be moved yet, and she couldn't argue with that.

'I should be able to stay there tomorrow night,' she said, for the umpteenth time, but he just leant back in his chair, Rufus curled up on his lap, and raised an eyebrow, his eyes sceptical.

'What, on that mattress? You need to wash it first at the very least—or replace it. And anyway, there's Lola to think of. At least here it's reasonably sterile and she can stay as long as she needs to.'

She sighed. 'I suppose you're right, and she's fine in the kennel while she recovers, but I'll go back there tomorrow and carry on until I've finished, then we should be able to stay there.'

He gave her another of those looks. 'On a wet mattress.'

'Or a new one.' Although she couldn't really afford it…

'Or you could just stay here?'

'What, sleeping by her kennel?'

He hesitated for a moment, as if he was about to say something else, then shrugged. 'Or in the office. It makes sense, at least as long as she's got the suction drain. She looks wiped, and after you took her out when we got back she went straight back into her kennel and went to sleep again. She needs more time, Ellie, you know that. There's no rush, and if you're with her you can keep a better eye on her, and reassure her.'

He was right. Of course he was right, but she felt like she was imposing on him, taking advantage of his good nature, and he'd already done enough. More than enough. Starting with saving Lola's life…

'OK. Just until Monday, though. That should give me time to get a replacement mattress from somewhere, and get everything clean.'

'We should be able to make some decent progress on it tomorrow,' he said then, taking her completely by surprise, and she stared at him.

'We?'

He frowned. 'Well—yes. I said I'd help.'

'You said you'd help *today*. I can't ask you to do that—'

'You didn't ask. I offered. And anyway,' he added with a grin, 'I'm trying to convince you I'm a decent human being so you'll take the job.'

She stared at him blankly. 'What job?'

Hugo did a mild double-take. 'The one I offered you this morning?'

Her heart thudded against her ribs. 'That was a serious job offer?'

'What did you think it was?'

She blinked and looked away. 'Uh—I don't know. I didn't realise you meant it.' And then she looked back and met his eyes, sincere and oddly intent. 'You seriously want me?'

Her words hit him like an express train, and he realised they were true—in every sense.

His heart thudded against his ribs, and he swallowed the sudden lump in his throat. 'Yes, I want you,' he said honestly. 'I need you.' And as he added that, he realised it, too, was true in every sense.

He ignored the thrashing of his pulse as he forced himself to hold her searching eyes. 'I desperately need another vet,' he said, to himself as much as to her. 'I think last night and this morning were a pretty good interview, Jim Harkness couldn't pile enough praise on your head—what else is there to think about?'

Apart from the fact that every time he caught the waft of scent from her body his gut tightened, every time she smiled or frowned or scraped that unruly tendril of dark hair back out of her incredible green eyes he wanted to kiss her—

He looked away, unable to hold that steady gaze for another second, not knowing what she might read in his eyes. He'd been told more than once that he'd be a lousy poker player.

'Can I think about it? I'm not sure I'm ready to commit to anything permanent yet. It's all been a bit sudden.'

He made himself meet her eyes again. 'Sure. I don't suppose you want to locum while you think?'

He held his breath while she hesitated, and then she nodded slowly. 'OK. Just for a while, until I decide what I'm doing with my life, and Lola's a bit better.'

That sounded a hugely sensible idea, and it meant neither of them would be committed to what already felt like a complicated relationship, at least on his side. And that was the last thing he needed. Thank goodness he hadn't offered her the flat. He'd been so close to it just now. He allowed himself to breathe again and hauled out a smile.

'Excellent. I think that calls for a celebration. How about a takeaway? I'll let you choose.'

By the end of the next day the upstairs was cleaned, the mattress included, and the bathroom had been scrubbed within an inch of its life, and with the windows open and a lovely fresh breeze blowing through the house everything was drying nicely.

'Better?'

She smiled at him and laughed. 'Much better. So, so much better. I don't know how to thank you, Hugo. You've been amazing.'

He chuckled softly and turned away before he did something stupid like haul her into his arms and kiss that smiling mouth.

'I had to do something to keep you on board,' he said lightly, and then picked up the carpet shampooer. 'I'll put this lot in the car while you shut the windows, and then we need to get back to the dogs. I think Lola's drain's probably ready to come out now, but I want to have a proper look at her first.'

'If she's OK and you've got a crate I can borrow, she and I can stay here tonight now.'

He frowned. 'Really? You've got no food, the mattress is still damp—what's the rush? And anyway, Lola isn't out of the woods yet, she'll need cage rest for another two weeks and you're working tomorrow, so you might as well be there or you'll have to move her backwards and forwards, which won't be comfortable for her. Besides, I've got a lasagne thawing and I can't eat it all.'

His logic was unassailable, but she still felt as if she was taking advantage. Plus, she was worried about the bill for Lola's in-patient treatment. All of it, really, because she'd taken out insurance for her after her abscess, and that wasn't yet a month. And anything in the first month was excluded, as he'd pointed out.

She thought about that all the way back, and as soon as they were in and the dogs were fed, she tackled him about it.

'You need to bill me for Lola's treatment and her care,' she said, and he raised an eyebrow and smiled.

'I think we've gone a little past that now, don't you?'

She frowned. 'But—'

'No buts. We'll be horrendously busy tomorrow morning with all the people who've hung on over the weekend so they didn't have to pay the out-of-hours rate, on top of an already full clinic, so I'll well and truly be getting my own back. And anyway, you're doing most of the caring, and we're hardly short of kennel space.'

He wasn't going to budge, she could tell that

just from the look he gave her, but there was still room to negotiate.

'On one condition,' she said firmly. 'I don't want the standard locum rate, I want you to work out what you'd pay for a full-time vet, divide it by the number of hours they'd work, and pay me that pro-rata. And I'll pay her bill. You can give me a staff discount if it makes you feel better.'

One eyebrow quirked up. 'You're cheating yourself.'

'No, I'm just not cheating *you.* I don't need to rip you off, I just need to earn enough to live on. Take it or leave it.'

'And if I say no?'

'Then you're a vet down tomorrow.'

He held her eyes, then a slow smile tipped his mouth at one side, and he nodded, and she felt the tension seep out of her. 'You're a very stubborn person, do you know that?' he said mildly, and then with a little shake of his head and a tiny huff of laughter, he looked down at Lola, resting in her kennel and watching them.

'We need to check that drain,' he said, and closed the subject.

CHAPTER THREE

THERE WAS NO 'easing in gently' or giving her the simple stuff on Monday morning. After an early start to sort Lola out, she was straight in with a dog spay, a cat castrate and then a cruciate repair on a terrier who'd snapped a ligament in his knee joint.

Kerry must have given him a heads up on that, she realised, as he stuck his head out of his consulting room.

'I think he probably needs a lateral suture. Are you happy to do that?'

'Sure. I've done it before—I've got an ortho certificate.'

He nodded. 'Good. Kerry'll give you a hand, help you find what you need and assist. Shout if you run into any issues.'

'Will do.'

She didn't, to her relief, and after she'd finished the operation and they'd X-rayed him and Ellie was confident the joint was going to be stable, she and Kerry put him into a small kennel cage in the area where Lola was lying, looking bored.

At least her drain was out and her leg was healing nicely. It would still take a good while, but she'd be left with a fine, neat scar and a functional leg, thanks to Hugo.

She was relieved by that. Poor Lola had had enough to deal with. 'Hello, sweetie,' she said, giving her dog a little tickle through the bars, but there wasn't time for more, even though Lola was pleading and pawing at the door.

'I'll take her out for a wee,' Kerry said, and Ellie left them to it and went to see if there were any more consults she could help with.

She was on the last one, a little spaniel puppy called Mr Wiggles in for his second vaccinations, when the door at the back opened and Hugo stuck his head round.

'I hear there's a puppy,' he said with a grin, and he came in and gave the wiggly little pup a cuddle while she drew up his vaccinations.

He obviously knew the owner, and they chatted while she gave him the injection.

'Oh, you're such a good boy,' Ellie said, ruffling his long floppy ears, and he wiggled and licked her.

'They're so forgiving,' his owner said with a laugh, and carried the puppy out, leaving her alone with Hugo.

'So how's it been?'

'Busy? Good? Let me fill this in and we can talk about it.'

'Tell me over lunch, I'll make you a coffee,' he said, and she glanced up at the clock. Half past one, and consults started again at two.

'Thanks,' she said, and he left her to it. By the time she emerged three minutes later there was a coffee and a sandwich waiting for her in the kitchen, and she took it into the office and sat down with him.

'So, tell me all about your morning. How did you get on?'

'All right, I think. The spay and castrate were routine, and the cruciate repair seems stable.'

'Yeah, I had a look. Nice tidy job.'

It had been and she didn't really need his praise, but nevertheless it was good to hear, and she felt a silly little glow of pride. What a contrast to Craig, still bitter because she'd dumped him ten years ago.

Hugo, on the other hand, seemed like a genuinely decent human being. To date he'd been nothing but generous towards her, and she owed it to him to do her best in return.

'What are you doing tonight?' he asked, and she swallowed her bite of sandwich and shrugged.

'Moving my stuff into the house, I guess. Taking Lola home with me, settling her in, buying some food—is it OK if I borrow a crate for a while?'

Hugo frowned. 'Ellie, you're welcome to a crate, but I don't think she's ready yet. She can't jump into the car, she can't do steps, she has to be on cage rest—I've been thinking, why don't you keep her in the kennel here and move into the flat upstairs till she's better?'

She stared at him. 'Hugo, you—I can't just move into your flat, it's ridiculous!'

'Not *my* flat,' he said hastily. 'There's another one, at the top. I'll show you later. I'm assuming you'd bring Lola to work every day anyway, wouldn't you?'

'Well, yes, if that's OK, but—'

'That's fine, then. She can lie here in the crate in the day for a change of scenery, and she can go back in the kennel at night. She'll have plenty of company, lots going on, you'll be able to keep an eye on her, and it won't stress the wound.'

She stared at him, slightly stunned. 'But—I thought you'd want us out of the way?'

'You're not in the way. And she's a sweetheart, she's no trouble. The flat's fully equipped, so you'll only need clothes and anything else you might want, so after we shut up shop I'll give you a hand to empty your car, and you can sort out what you want up there and put the rest in the store room, if you like?'

Did she like? She wasn't sure. He'd done so much for her, and being independent was hard-wired into her DNA, but nevertheless it seemed churlish to refuse his help after he'd already been so generous. And then there was the question of the rent, but she had no choice really while Lola was so immobile, she knew that. She just hoped she could afford it.

'Thanks for the offer, but I've got plenty of room for my things at the house, if you don't mind me leaving Lola here while I go and dump them?' she said, and he got to his feet.

'Sure. We can sort out the details later,' he said, drained the last of his coffee and headed out, and then Kerry came in, followed by Jean, the practice manager.

'Ah, Ellie, I need your bank details and all the other HR stuff for the records,' Jean said to her as she stood up to follow Hugo out. 'Not urgently, but when you can?'

'Sure. I've got to empty my car later, it's all in there. I'll give it to you tomorrow if that's OK?'

'That's fine. It's good to have you here, by the way,' she added. 'Hugo's been struggling for too long, and with our only other full-time vet off on maternity leave it's been ridiculous, so we're all really relieved that you turned up when you did.'

'I'm only locuming,' she said, feeling the net of commitment tightening around her, and Jean smiled knowingly.

'So he tells me, but you're still very welcome.'

And now she felt guilty for refusing to consider a permanent job.

Although the door to that was also still ajar…

As soon as she'd finished for the day she fed Lola and let her out, then put her away again and headed for the house.

It was the first time she'd been in it alone since Lola's accident, and she stood for a moment, listening to the silence.

Would it ever feel like home?

Weird thought. She'd never lived in a home that she owned, but it still felt like someone else's. Moving in might help, but Hugo of course had had a view about that and the moment Lola's leg was healed enough she'd be here like a shot.

She ferried all her belongings into the house, dumped them on the floor and stared at the pathetically small pile. It was everything she owned, but now she had a permanent base—

Did she want it to be that? Not necessarily. It didn't need to be, although apparently it could be, if Hugo had his way.

Did she want to take the job he'd offered, live here in Yoxburgh, start to put down new roots in a place she'd always loved but never really known?

A bit of her—the bit she didn't trust, because it had shown pretty lousy judgement in the past—said yes. The rest, the bit that had told Craig exactly where to stick his job, said no.

She didn't know enough about Hugo.

Yes, he'd been kind, yes, he'd been highly spoken of by her old boss, but what would he be like to work with? Fair, definitely, she was sure of that, but it all seemed too easy, and she didn't trust 'easy'. Not now, after all that had happened. And another job going wrong, if it did, would firmly put the kibosh on her CV. No. She'd locum for him, but that was it. She really, really wasn't ready to commit herself again so soon, and especially not to someone as charming as Hugo. She couldn't trust it. Couldn't trust *him,* whatever Jim had said.

She went through the pile of bags, pulled out the things she might need, stacked the rest under the stairs and then headed back to the practice with—not dread, exactly, but reluctance. She knew it made sense, she knew Lola couldn't easily be moved backwards and forwards yet, but right now she felt so dislocated that she was desperate for a home of her own.

And she was going to be living in Hugo's flat. Well, not *his* exactly, but as good as. Was that a good idea? It didn't sound like it, but he was frankly too kind for his own good and she owed him so much already that she didn't really want to put on him any more. But she felt stressed and a bit cornered, and if it hadn't been for Lola…

If it hadn't been for Lola she'd still be working

with the odious Craig, but she wasn't, and Lola had to come first.

She drove into the car park just as Hugo was parking his car, and he got out and waved a shopping bag at her.

'Supper,' he said, and she felt another wave of guilt to add to the stress.

'Hugo, you should have sent me a shopping list! I didn't even think about food, but I can't keep sponging off you.'

'Don't be ridiculous.'

He closed the gates and locked them, and she followed him in through the staff entrance, bags in hand.

'Right, I'll just get Rufus and we'll take all this up and go and eat.'

'What about Lola?'

'She's fine, I checked on her before I went out. She's sleeping and there's a camera so we can keep an eye on her on my phone. Let's get this food cooked. I'm starving.'

He let Rufus out of his crate and she followed them up what must once have been the wide main stairs of the house, past a glorious stained glass window and onto a large, open landing with a high ceiling and ornate cornicing. The flat was much bigger than she'd imagined, certainly bigger than the one she'd recently vacated, thanks to Craig, and significantly nicer. Much bigger than her house, too, but that wasn't difficult.

His bedroom door was open just enough to see a large sleigh bed, the duvet neatly turned back to air. She dragged her eyes and imagination off it and followed him into the kitchen, light and bright and spotlessly clean, with a range of integrated appliances and a table by the window.

'Right, food,' he said, and unloaded the shopping. 'Are you OK with fish pie?'

Her stomach rumbled, and he chuckled. 'I'll take that as a yes.' He put the oven on to heat, and she leant against the worktop and tried not to watch him as he removed the film from the top of the ready meal and put it in the oven.

'This is a lovely flat,' she said, and he smiled.

'It is, isn't it? I've redecorated it and refitted the kitchen and bathroom, but I don't spend nearly enough time in it. I'll show you the other one now while the food heats, if you like?'

'Sure.'

They went through a door off his hallway, onto the landing of what must have been the old back stairs. She followed him up into a much smaller but equally well-presented space, with a double bedroom, a shower room, a small but well-equipped kitchen and a welcoming living room, all with sloping ceilings at the sides making it seem cosy and intimate. And homely.

She stood in the dormer window of the sitting room looking down into the garden and felt him move to stand behind her.

'You can see the sea from here,' he murmured, pointing towards the gap between the houses. 'Look along my finger.'

She did, leaning altogether too close to him to look and feeling the brush of the soft hairs on his forearm teasing her cheek and making it tingle.

'Found it? It's only a glimpse.'

She had, the line of the horizon peeping through the rooftops, but it wasn't nearly as fascinating as the scent drifting off his body, an intoxicating combination of citrus and the rich, warm note of musk from his skin, and her cheek was still tingling.

'Yes, I can see it,' she murmured, and he dropped his arm so she could breathe again.

'So what do you think?'

She thought he smelt more delicious than a man had any right to smell, but she put the thought firmly out of her mind. She inched away from him and sucked in a quiet breath.

'It's lovely. Perfect,' she added, and felt some of the stress drain away.

'Tell me if you think it would be any kind of incentive to a new vet. I was thinking of putting it in the advert.'

Her eyes widened. 'Goodness, yes, I would have thought anyone would be tempted by it, especially as you live here, too, so it means they don't have all the responsibility for the practice at night. I found that quite challenging, sometimes, and I was always the first person to any emergency, of course.'

He laughed and moved away. 'Yes, I know how that works,' he said, and headed towards the door. 'Come on, let's go and have our meal, then you can settle in.'

'We need to talk about rent,' she said, and he turned back to her with a frown.

'Rent? What rent?'

'For the flat.'

He gave a soft huff of laughter and shook his head slowly. 'There is no rent, Ellie. If it goes with the job, it goes with the job. And right now, you're doing the job. End of.'

Feeling slightly stunned and a lot relieved, Ellie followed him back down.

The fish pie was delicious, and after they'd eaten it he made them coffee and picked the mugs up.

'Let's go and sit down somewhere comfortable,' he said, and led her to the sitting room, with a beautiful marble fireplace and the same original plaster cornicing. It must have been a very grand house in its day.

Not that it wasn't grand now, but in a more relaxed way—especially since Rufus had made himself at home on the sofa.

'This is a beautiful room,' she said, and he smiled.

'It is, isn't it? I really should spend more time in here.'

She settled herself into what had to be the comfiest sofa in the world and cradled the mug in her hands.

'So how come you're a vet?' she asked, partly out of curiosity and partly to fill the silence, and he gave a soft grunt.

'Oh—long story.'

'I've got time. And you've had to put up with mine.'

She looked at him and he smiled, but it didn't reach his eyes and he looked away before she did.

'Well, you asked, so here goes.' He hesitated for a moment, then started to speak, his voice flat and matter-of-fact.

'My father was a consultant surgeon at Addenbrooke's in Cambridge, my mother was a GP until I came along, then she stayed at home and looked after me and did all the admin for his private work. They got a dog, because I nagged, and every time she needed the vet I went along, and I was interested. I told my father I wanted to be a vet like my godfather Peter, and he said no. Be a doctor. If you're a vet, you'll spend all your time killing things. If you're a doctor, you'll be saving lives.'

Ellie stared at him, stunned. 'We save lives. We save lives every single day!'

'I know. That's what I told him, and I told him

lots of people die, doctors or no doctors, but looking back I think he didn't want me to be a vet because he regarded it as inferior. And then our dog got sick, and our vet couldn't save her, and she was put to sleep—which just proved his point.'

'So why *aren't* you a doctor?'

'Because I've never wanted to be. Peter's influence, probably, and because I've always loved animals. This was his practice, and I used to love it when we stayed here and I could spend time with his menagerie. And then when I was ten, Mum was diagnosed with cancer, and Dad had a heart attack. They inserted a stent, put him on all the drugs, and he was fine and she was responding well to the chemo, but then two years later she was told it had spread and it was terminal, and a week later he had another massive heart attack and died.'

She sucked in a breath, her heart aching for the boy he'd been. 'Oh, Hugo. I'm so sorry. How old were you?'

'Twelve. But in a way it proved me right, because the doctors couldn't save him, any more than they could save my mother. She died two years after him, when I was fourteen, and I spent a lot of time here with Peter and Sally during her last few months. Mum had made Peter my legal guardian when she knew she was dying, and they took me in and welcomed me with open arms. They'd never had children, and Peter would have been a brilliant father. He *was* a brilliant father, and Sally was a wonderful mother figure, so kind, so understanding. And after Mum died, I was horrible to them.'

'Horrible?'

He gave a tiny huff of laughter. 'Yeah. I was fourteen, and I was an orphan. That's all I could hear, that word, and nothing could take it away. I was utterly broken with grief and anger, but they understood why, and they gave me the little flat. I still ate with them, lived with them, really, but it became my bolt-hole, my sanctuary, and it saved my sanity because I had a private space to grieve in and to come to terms with what was now my life.'

Her eyes welled over and she blinked to clear them. 'That must have been so hard.'

'It was, but I left my old school and went to one in Woodbridge, and I never told anyone there that my parents were dead, so I didn't have to deal with their sympathy, which made it easier. Peter took me under his wing, gave me his time unstintingly, and when I'd got over the initial trauma, he showed me everything he could. He had me doing stuff in the practice every holiday, and when that got boring he fixed me up with some farmers so I could learn about sheep and cattle, then he sent me off to a stable yard where I spent a glorious summer mucking out the horses and learning how to handle them, and all the time he was keeping me on target in school, making sure I got the grades I needed.'

He threw her a wry smile. 'Not that he had to push me, I was all the way there myself, but then they supported me through uni until I got my first job in a mixed practice, then he took me on himself when I decided I wanted to specialise in companion animals. He mentored me, taught me everything he knew, and when he retired eight years ago at sixty I bought him out. I'd moved back into the little flat when I started work here, and I lived in it until Peter and Sally moved out, and then I renovated this one, moved into it and did up the little one.'

'So it really is home to you,' she said, and he nodded.

'Oh, yes, absolutely. This place has been a life-saver, one way or another, and it's been my home and sanctuary for the last twenty-five years.'

So he was thirty-nine, and he'd been a year younger than she was when he'd bought the practice. There was no way she could even dream of doing that.

'It feels like it wraps itself round you,' she said softly.

'It always did. I think it was their love that did that. I owe them everything, him and Sally, and my parents. They left their estate in trust for me until I was twenty-five, which meant I was able to buy the practice, but—yeah, everything I am today, I owe to Peter. He literally saved my life and gave me a reason to go on, and I owe him more than I can ever say.'

'He sounds pretty special,' she said softly after a long pause. 'You were lucky to have him as a father figure.'

'I was. I've been so, so lucky to have them both in my life, and without them there's no way I'd be here doing the job I love.'

'And Jim? How did you end up there?'

'Rotation via college. Peter knew him, though, so maybe that was another string he pulled, but he never said so. It wouldn't surprise me. They've stuck by me through thick and thin, and some of it's been pretty tough.'

He drew in a long, slow breath and turned to look at her, and she knew from the shield that had come down over his eyes that there was something else that he wasn't telling her.

'So that's me,' he said, done with the confessions. 'How about you? Why are you a vet?'

She held his eyes for a long moment, then gave him a strange little smile and looked away.

'Good question. I don't really know the answer. It just sort of...evolved. I wasn't sure it was what I wanted, but there was nothing else that was ever on my radar, and I had to do something.'

'Had to?' he asked, probing a little.

'Well—yes. I had to earn a living, but I needed

a career that would give me job satisfaction, I was bright, I loved animals—it just seemed a bit obvious really.'

'But?'

She shrugged. 'But I was never really sure. I found it all a bit intimidating, but my mother was very keen that I should make the best of myself and take whatever opportunities were presented to me.'

My mother?

'What did your father think?' he asked, probing a little.

She gave a hollow little laugh that spoke volumes. 'I have no idea. He left my mother when I was little and I haven't seen him since, so I've never had a father figure.'

That shocked him. 'You've never seen him?'

'No, and there's never been any father figure in my life. You don't know how lucky you are.'

'Oh, I do. Believe me, I do. So how did your mum cope?'

'I don't know. It must have been tough. She had to work hard to support and house us on her own. There were times when it was really hard, and after all she put into it, I couldn't let her down.'

'And if she hadn't been like that?'

'Then maybe I would have found something else to do, something less challenging, less complicated, less—difficult.'

That was odd. 'Difficult?'

She looked at him, then away again, a slightly twisted smile on her lips. ‘Difficult. Yes, we save lives, but as your father said, we also take them, and we have to break a lot of bad news. I always find that hard. It breaks their hearts, and—I don’t know, sometimes there just seem to be days when you have to do it over and over, and it drains you.’

‘But not as much as watching animals suffer because the owners, often for good reason, can’t bear to let them go. I watched my mother die of cancer, and I wouldn’t wish that on anyone, human or animal.’

She nodded slowly. ‘Yes, I get that, and I absolutely agree. It’s a privilege to be able to spare them that, but—then you get a dog like Lola, otherwise fit and healthy, who can easily be saved with a simple operation and some antibiotics, and you have to put it to sleep, because you can’t just take them all in or you’d end up running an animal shelter.’

‘But you took Lola.’

She looked down at Rufus between them, and he watched a tear slide down her cheek as she stroked him gently.

‘Yes, I did, and I’d do it again, but look where it got us both. And what if it happens again? What if there’s another Lola? When do you stop?’

He reached out and put his hand over hers and gave her fingers a little squeeze, then left it there, his thumb absently stroking the back of her hand.

'There'll always be another Lola. That's how I got Rufus. Elderly owner, unaffordable bill, energetic pup she couldn't cope with. Her kids had bought him for her to cheer her up after her husband died, but she wasn't ready for it and she couldn't cope with a puppy. And her family weren't able to take him on, because they all worked full-time, and they couldn't pay the bill either, so I did what you did, I took him on.'

She looked up and met his eyes, her lips tilting in a sad little smile that made something inside him ache to comfort her.

'We're a right pair, aren't we?' she said, and he chuckled.

'You could say that,' he said, and gave her fingers another quick squeeze and retrieved his hand before it got too used to holding hers. 'And talking of dogs, we need to take them both out, and then you need to settle in.'

She followed him down the stairs, and while he took Rufus in the garden she went into the kennel area and found Lola fast asleep.

'Lola? Wake up, sweetie,' she murmured.

She opened the kennel door, and Lola lifted her head and stared at her, and she took the cone off and stroked her gently. 'Come on, poppet, let's take you out in the garden and then put you back to bed. We've got another busy day tomorrow and I need some sleep.'

They went out, and after Rufus had sniffed Lola and she'd returned the favour, she bopped down for her wee and then led Ellie back inside and went straight into her kennel and lay down.

He's right, Ellie thought. *She's not ready for anything other than rest right now.* She sat with her for a while until Hugo came in, and he crouched down beside her, the tantalising waft of warm male body drifting over her again as he gave Lola a gentle stroke.

'She's a good girl,' he murmured, and she swallowed hard.

'She is—and you were absolutely right, she's not ready for anything other than lying here and recovering. Thank you for letting me use the flat while that happens.'

'You're welcome. Shout if you need anything, you know where I am.' His mouth tilted in a slight smile, and after a second he straightened up. 'I'll take your bags up for you. See you tomorrow. Sleep well.'

'You, too—and thank you.'

His mouth tipped again into that smile she was getting all too fond of, and he went upstairs with Rufus, taking his warmth away but leaving the faint lingering trace of his scent that teased her senses and made her think things she really, really shouldn't. Not if she wanted to keep her sanity.

She put the cone back on Lola, changed her

water and settled her for the night before heading up the back stairs, past the door that led to his flat, on up the second flight to her temporary home.

At least the bed was made, presumably in readiness for a guest, and she was more than ready to crawl into it and find some oblivion. He'd put her bags on the chest of drawers, and she found her wash things and cleaned her teeth, then lay down in the welcoming, comfy bed, desperate for sleep and yet wide awake, her thoughts tumbling.

Yet again, Hugo had come riding to the rescue. Yes, sure, he needed a vet and if she'd taken Lola home, she could only have worked restricted hours for a while, so he might have had a vested interest, and of course there was the permanent job he kept dangling in front of her like a nice juicy carrot.

But she knew enough about Hugo now to realise that his offer might simply have been an act of kindness. Did he really need another vet? Jean had said someone was on maternity leave. Did he know that she wasn't coming back? Or coming back part-time? Or was it just Hugo being Hugo…?

She rolled onto her side with a little growl of frustration, tugged the pillow into the crook of her neck and shut her eyes firmly.

One day at a time. Starting with tomorrow.

CHAPTER FOUR

ANY DOUBTS SHE might have had about Hugo's motivation vanished the next morning. By the time she'd dealt with Lola and was ready to start it was a quarter to eight, but there were already three cars in the car park, and she could hear Hugo's voice rattling off instructions in the background.

She followed the sound and found him surrounded by nurses, all working furiously on a puppy. Her little spaniel puppy of yesterday, Mr Wiggles.

'Anything I can do?' she asked, and he shook his head.

'No, short of teaching puppies not to eat stuff they shouldn't. Right, let's open him up and find out what's going on. Ellie, could you pick up the consults, please? I'm going to be tied up for a bit.'

'Sure.'

She left them to it, and for the next half hour she did mostly routine things—until it all hit the fan with Chester, a two-year-old Dalmatian that had eaten chewing gum.

His owner was distraught. 'I wasn't sure if it mattered, but I looked it up on the Internet and I thought I ought to bring him in. He hadn't wanted to go for his walk, and then he seemed floppy and started to vomit, and a bit of gum came up, and then I saw the pot lying on the floor. He must have got it off the worktop—'

'How much was in the pot?'

'About a third? I don't know. I brought it to show you.'

She pulled out a small pot, her hands shaking, and Ellie's heart sank. Sugar-free gum with xylitol—and a third of the pot?

'OK, I'm going to have to admit him and get him on a glucose drip fast because his body thinks he's had a lot of sugar and will be pumping out insulin. Get Reception to give you a consent form to sign, and I'll get the drip in now, but don't worry, I think we've got him in time.'

She scooped the floppy dog up and carried him quickly out to the prep room. 'Can anyone help me, please? I've got a dog who's ingested xylitol.'

Kerry detached herself from the puppy group and came over. 'I'll warm the dextrose. Can you get a line in?'

'Sure.' She shaved his front leg, slid in the cannula, withdrew bloods for analysis and flushed the line, and by the time she'd done that and given him a bolus of dextrose to kickstart his blood sugar recovery, the bag of dextrose was warmed and she hung the drip up and checked the blood results as soon as they came up, with Kerry monitoring him constantly.

His glucose levels had been at rock bottom, but he was slowly starting to wake up, to her relief.

Then Hugo arrived at her side, a brush of warmth against her arm, sending distracting tingles through her body.

'How's he doing?'

Focus!

'OK, I think. We might just have caught it in time. Do you have any hepatoprotectant, in case his liver's affected?'

'Yes, I'll get you some. Kerry, what does he weigh?'

'He was twenty-six point four kg last time he was weighed,' Kerry said promptly, and Hugo nodded and disappeared, coming back a minute later with the drug.

'So how's Mr Wiggles?' she asked as they worked, and he rolled his eyes.

'Better without a rubber toy in his gut.'

'What? How on earth did he swallow that?'

'No idea. It's a special skill dogs have. Do you want me to update Chester's owner on how he's doing?'

'Sure, if you've got time. I'm just going to check his bloods again, but I think he needs hospitalising. He's not out of the woods yet. He's going to need his glucose and liver enzymes monitored hourly for seventy-two hours.'

He gave her a wry smile. 'I'll go and break the news. I'm sure Mrs Grey will be delighted.'

Mrs Grey *was* delighted. Not by the fact that she'd have to drive him to the specialist centre, but because he was still alive and they'd hopefully managed to start his treatment in time.

She sat and waited for an hour until they were sure he was stable, then Hugo carried him out to the car for her.

'Thank you, Hugo. And please thank Ellie for me,' she said. 'She was so lovely to me, so quick and efficient and yet she still found time to be kind. I'm so, so grateful to you all.'

'I'll pass it on,' he said, and he went back inside. She was in consults again, and he checked on Mr Wiggles before he started his next op, a routine spay that had already been delayed two hours.

Thank God for Ellie. If he hadn't been sure of her before, he was now. He needed her in his practice. He just wasn't sure how to persuade her. Maybe Mrs Grey's message would do the trick…

The rest of the day didn't get any better.

Apart from a snatched biscuit, Ellie hadn't eaten since breakfast and by six she was running on adrenaline alone.

She said goodbye to her last client with a sigh of relief, and went out to Reception.

'Right, that's me done for the day, unless you've got anything else that's come in?' she said to Jean.

'No, we're done. Hugo's last client didn't turn up, so he's in the office and I'm going to lock the door.'

'Thank goodness for that,' she said. 'I can't believe it's still Tuesday.'

But before Jean could get to the door, a woman burst in.

'Where's Hugo? Nell's had a dreadful accident—'

'Find him, I'll go,' Ellie said to Jean without hesitation, and she ran out with the woman and found an elderly Labrador lying in the back of a car, shaking and whimpering, one leg bent at an ominous angle.

'I was bringing her to Hugo to put to sleep because of her cancer, but she slipped off the ramp getting into the car and…'

She broke off, sobbing, and Ellie gave her a quick hug. 'I'll go and get the drugs and find Hugo. Don't worry, I'll be really quick. You stay with her.'

She ran back in and found Hugo on his way out to them.

'What's up with Nell?' he asked.

'Fractured femur. She slipped getting in the car.'

He swore. 'I'll get the stuff. Can you help, please?'

It wasn't really a question that needed answering. They went out together, and found Nell's owner sitting under the tailgate by her head, stroking her side, her face grief-stricken, and she looked up at Hugo through eyes filled with tears.

'Hugo, this is all my fault, please don't let her hurt any more,' she said, and he hugged her briefly.

'Don't worry, Jenny, it'll be quick and I'll be very gentle.'

She moved out of the way, and he leant into the car.

'Hello, sweetheart,' he murmured tenderly, stroking Nell's head, and the dog looked up at him with pleading eyes. 'It's OK, Nell, it's all going to be OK, good girl,' he said, his voice low and soothing, and as soon as Ellie had clipped the little area of hair on her front leg and pressed her thumb on the vein to raise it, he took the syringe and slid in the needle, and as Ellie stepped out of the way, Nell's head sank down and she gave a quiet sigh.

'There we go, Nell,' he crooned softly, stroking her head with gentle fingers. 'It's all over now.' He put the stethoscope on her chest to listen to her heart, then turned to Jenny. 'She's gone now,' he said quietly, and stroked the old dog's head again tenderly as he straightened up.

'It's my fault,' she said, sobbing and cradling Nell's lolling head against her. 'I should have listened to you before…'

'You weren't to know she'd slip like that,' Hugo said, his voice gentle, one hand rubbing her shoulder to comfort her. 'Will you be OK to drive home?'

She nodded. 'I will be now. Thank you so much.' She sniffed and straightened up, visibly pulling herself together. 'Um—I need to pay you.'

'Don't worry about that now. Do you still want her cremated?'

'Please. That would be so kind, Hugo. We've buried the others but since I lost George…'

He squeezed her shoulder. 'It's no problem. You take care. I'll be in touch.'

Hugo lifted Nell out of the car as gently as he would an injured child, her owner kissed her goodbye and he carried her into the back of the practice while Ellie held Jenny as she sobbed, her own eyes filling with tears.

She felt Jenny drag in a huge breath and straighten up, swiping at her eyes and fumbling for a tissue.

'Are you going to be OK?' Ellie asked her.

Her smile was sad, but her face was calmer. 'I will be. It's just the shock. She was our fifth dog, and I don't know why we kept doing it, setting ourselves up for heartache. I don't know why anyone does it.'

'Because we love them, and they bring us so much joy in their short lives. Just try and remember the good times.'

'I will, but I'll never forgive myself. Since George died she's always been by my side, and the guilt will live with me for ever. She was my best friend in my darkest hours, and I let her down…'

'No, you didn't, it was an accident. You loved her till the end, and she knew that. Don't worry, we'll take good care of her and Hugo will give you a call about her ashes.'

'Thank you,' she said, and as she drove away Ellie watched her go, tears blurring her view.

She turned and went back inside, and walked straight into Hugo's arms. They wrapped around her like a protective cocoon, and she rested her head against his shoulder for a moment, soaking up his warmth and strength. She could have stayed there for ever, breathing in the scent of his body, listening to the steady, reassuring thud of his heart beneath her ear.

'You OK?' he murmured softly, and she nodded and straightened up, and he gave her shoulders a quick squeeze before letting her go.

She followed him into the prep room where Nell was lying on the table, and she walked over to her and stroked her head tenderly. 'Poor Nell. Such a sad end. You know I hate it, we were talking about it last night, but when it's like that…'

He nodded. 'I know. I'm just sorry Jenny didn't let me do it the last time she was here and then this wouldn't have happened.'

'She told me Nell was her best friend and she let her down. She said she'll never forgive herself.'

'It's always easy to be wise after the event. They've listened to advice in the past, but maybe Nell was the last link to George. I wonder if she'll get another.'

Ellie looked down at Nell and stroked her again. 'I expect she will, the house will seem awfully empty without a dog. She said they've had five.'

'They have. I've known them all.'

She studied his face, searching his eyes as he held her gaze. There was something in his eyes, something dark and—angry? No, not angry. More…

'There's something else.'

He gave a soft laugh that wasn't a laugh at all, and looked away. 'You don't miss much, do you?' he murmured, then went on, 'My mother had a pathological fracture of her femur—she stumbled in the garden and it went. Luckily I was there with her. They took her to hospital and pinned it, then she moved to a hospice and never went home again. That was when I came to live with Peter and Sally. So—yeah, pathological fractures are a bit of a sore point.'

She could see why. How traumatic for a fourteen-year-old to witness that. 'You hid it well from Jenny.'

He shrugged. 'That's what we do. We keep our own feelings under wraps, and manage theirs. And sometimes it's harder than others. Nell was a lovely dog. I was very fond of her, and so was Jenny, but I understand how hard it is to say goodbye. It's a difficult decision. Grief is always difficult, but this just made it a whole lot harder for them both. And yet we do it to ourselves over and over again,' he added quietly, looking down at Rufus who was leaning devotedly against his leg as if he knew he needed comfort.

He reached down and Rufus licked his hand, and she smiled round the lump in her throat.

He straightened up, his eyes glittering a little before he turned away. 'I need to take Nell to the cremation guy, and I've got a couple of others to drop off as well. If you're not busy you could come with me?'

She stared at his back, trying to work out if he wanted her there or not. Should she go?

Probably, but Lola had had a boring day in her kennel, and Rufus had been in the office all day. 'Is it far?'

'About twenty minutes away.'

She hesitated again. 'Wouldn't it be better if I stayed with the dogs? And I need to go and buy some food.'

'Do that tomorrow. I've got stuff in my fridge that needs eating—I could knock us up something when I get back?'

She was so tempted, partly because of Nell and how it had affected him, but—another meal eaten with him? That would make it the fifth night on the trot. Every night, in fact, since she'd arrived at the practice with Lola trying to bleed to death. And he hadn't turned *her* away, either. No wonder he looked exhausted. The man didn't know how to say no.

'It's not that hard to decide, is it?' he asked, a smile tugging at his lips, and she gave a little laugh.

'No, it's not that hard, but I'll cook. It's definitely my turn.'

'Well, use the food in my fridge or it'll turn up its toes. I shouldn't be more than an hour. I'll take Rufus, he likes a run in the car.'

While he loaded the car and set off, she removed Lola's cone and took her out into the garden briefly, and then fed her and sat beside her on the floor in the office, Lola's head on her lap and her good leg raised for a tummy rub.

The wound on her other one was healing nicely, thanks to Hugo. She chewed her lip and wondered how much her bill was going to be. She owed him so much for last Friday night, not to mention the inpatient fees, and every time she raised the subject Hugo brushed it aside.

She'd have to pin him down—or ask Jean. She'd do that tomorrow.

Lola rolled her head round and stared up at her. 'Yes, I will,' she said to her. 'I'll ask Jean tomorrow, but right now, sweetie, you need to go back in your kennel and I need to go and see what Hugo's got in his fridge.'

Lots, was the answer. Some chicken thighs with a short date, lots of fresh green veg, a small pot of crème fraiche, again with a short date, the remains of the parmesan he'd used on Friday night, and there was even a pot of basil growing on the windowsill.

She found dried herbs, stock cubes and olive oil in a cupboard near the hob and another rummage in the fridge came up with garlic and a small jar of sundried tomatoes.

She smiled. Excellent. She had everything she needed.

She'd just finished cooking when she heard his car pull up, and by the time she'd put the veg in the pan ready to steam and a pouch of rice in the microwave, she heard the door at the bottom of the stairs open.

Rufus arrived first, of course, rushing in to

greet her and sniff around for anything she might have dropped, followed by Hugo, also sniffing.

'Wow, what are you cooking? It smells amazing.'

'It is amazing, and it's also super easy and you just happened to have all the ingredients. I hope you weren't saving any of them for anything special?'

'No, nothing. So what is it?'

She felt him close, his breath teasing her cheek as he peered over her shoulder into the pan.

'It's vaguely Italian. For some ludicrous reason it's called Marry Me Chicken,' she said, turning her head as his eyes widened, and she gave a stifled laugh and turned away again, wishing she hadn't told him. 'Don't panic, that's not significant, it's just one of the few things I can cook.'

She heard a low chuckle. 'Well, if it tastes as good as it smells I can imagine why it got the name. How long will it be?'

'Three minutes? I just need to steam the veg.'

'I'll go and change. Dish up when it's ready, I won't be long.'

He walked into his bedroom, closed the door and leant on it, letting out a long, slow breath.

Yes, it smelt amazing, but so did she, and standing that close, the combination of the rich sauce and the drift of something tantalising from her hair had sent a shiver of something powerful and potent streaking through his body.

Three minutes? He'd need three hours in a cold shower to unravel that. But then again, Marry Me Chicken? Really?

In another world, at another time—but not here, not now. Not ever. Not since—

He felt his chest tighten and slammed the door on that thought, peeled off his clothes, dragged on a pair of jeans and a long-sleeved T and went back out to find she'd laid the table under the window and was about to dish up.

Good. He wouldn't need to make small talk.

'Thanks for your help with Nell,' he said, propping himself up against the worktop and folding his arms.

She looked slightly surprised at that. 'You don't need to thank me. And for what it's worth, if I was ever in any doubt about you genuinely needing another vet, it's gone. Today was crazy.'

'It was, and I was very grateful for your help. My job offer still stands, just so you know. Oh, and I have a message for you from Mrs Grey, she wanted me to thank you. She said you were very kind to her and really great with Chester. She was impressed. And he's doing fine so far. I rang and checked on the way back and his blood glucose level's picked up and he's stable now.'

'Good. We weren't sure how much he'd had, really, but I didn't want to take any chances.'

'No, very wise. Right, let's eat this, I'm starving,' he said, and he sat down with his plate and took a mouthful.

Wow. His taste buds all but cried with joy, and he gave up any attempt at small talk and scraped the plate clean. If he'd been on his own, he might even have licked it. Instead he swallowed and met her eyes.

'That is *the best* chicken dish I've ever tasted. I don't care what it's called, I want the recipe.'

She gave a tiny laugh and looked away, and he wasn't sure if her cheeks were turning a soft shade of pink or if it was just the heat from cooking. Whatever, he had to fight the urge to kiss her—

'Sure. I'll zap the link to your phone. There's enough left for you tomorrow.'

He swallowed. 'Excellent. And thank you.'

'You're welcome—and thank *you*. It was your food.'

His laugh sounded a little hollow. 'If you can do that with my ingredients, you can cook for me any time you want.'

This time her laugh was real. 'Don't push your luck. It's about the only thing I can cook apart from pasta and jacket potatoes. Right, I'll clear this lot up, and then I'd better get Lola settled for the night.'

'And I'd better take Rufus for a walk, and then I really need to do some admin. See you tomorrow?'

'Sure, since you clearly need me.'

Something flickered in his eyes for a second, and then he bent down and ruffled Rufus's ears again, her words hanging in the air between them.

'Yes, we need you,' he said, his voice oddly gruff. He pushed back his chair and headed for the door without meeting her eyes. 'Thanks again, Ellie. I'll see you in the morning. Rufus, come.'

Ellie stared after him, trying to work out what if anything had just happened there.

No. She was imagining it, trying to make something out of nothing. He was simply grateful for another pair of hands, and it was nothing more than that, however much she might want it to be.

And anyway, now wasn't the time. She had a new life to build, to find her place in the world now it had been turned upside down.

He'd be such a wonderful father...

And where had that thought come from? She'd barely met him and she was dreaming about his babies!

She felt a curious stab of longing, and stifled it. Getting tangled up with Hugo would be silly right now.

However much she wanted it…

* * *

How could it *be* so difficult?

She wasn't interested in him—or at least not in the job. She'd made that clear enough—and yet there was something that drew him relentlessly to her.

Why? She was a vet, and he needed a vet more than he needed anything else in the world right now, or his health would start to suffer and his practice would collapse. And that wouldn't help anyone. And even if he *was* interested in her, there was no way, not with the little he had to offer. Apart from the fact that his dedication to his job screwed up every relationship before it really got off the ground, like it had with Emma, he couldn't offer her anything like the relationship she deserved.

She needed someone kind, someone who was able to love her whole-heartedly. Someone who'd give her the family life she'd never had. And that wasn't him. Didn't stop him wanting her…

He swallowed hard. Time to start advertising again. Maybe if he chucked in the flat he might get a couple of decent candidates. With rents sky-rocketing and an uncertain housing market, free accommodation could be a winner. If he could get anyone else competent enough to do the job.

Someone as competent and capable and caring as Ellie…

Never going to happen.

'Come on, Rufus,' he said with a sigh, and he put the little dog on a lead and headed out of the door. A good brisk walk along the sea front would clear his head and sort it out.

Except he'd only got halfway to the gates when he realised there was a cardboard box outside them. Rufus tugged him towards it, and as he unlocked the gate and bent to open it he heard a distressed miaow coming from inside the box.

His heart sinking, he picked up the box carefully, went back inside, shut the confused Rufus in the office and went into a consulting room, closing the door behind him before he opened the lid in case the cat escaped.

There was no way the tiny little cat was going anywhere. She stared up at him, hugely pregnant, utterly exhausted and clearly in need of help. He lifted her out carefully and examined her, and as her abdomen went rigid with a contraction, he noticed a tiny paw protruding.

The kitten was still alive, the paw flexing slightly when he touched it, but it was clearly obstructed. And he didn't have much time. Damn.

He called Ellie and she picked up on the second ring.

'I've got a very pregnant cat in obstructed labour. Fancy some overtime?'

'Give me ten seconds to change and I'll come down.'

He hung up and carried the poor little cat

through to the prep room, laid her down, shaved her leg in readiness then put her back in the box and quickly got out all the things they'd need for a C section, then stripped and pulled on some scrubs. By the time he'd done that Ellie was there. She'd had the sense to put scrubs on, too, and they anaesthetised the little cat and opened her up and carefully eased out the kittens. Six were alive, and the seventh, the one that had been stuck and that he finally managed to free by easing it back, was borderline.

He took the borderline one and worked on it while Ellie rubbed the live ones and got them mewling and tucked them under a heat lamp, and then she took the limp, barely alive kitten from him and breathed into its mouth while he closed up the mother.

'How is he?' he asked.

'I think he's trying to breathe—yes, he's breathing!'

'Wow. I thought he wouldn't make it. I reckon he'd been stuck for ages, but I think we deserved some luck after Nell. But there you go, you win some, you lose some. Right, can you monitor mum while I finish closing, please? And then we need to get these babies snuggled up to her.'

She put the little kitten down with the others under the heat lamp, and turned back to the mother with a quiet groan.

'Problem?' he asked, and she shook her head.

'No, she seems OK at the moment, but it's going to be a long night and my bed's calling me already,' she said, and he gave a short laugh. Her bed was calling him, too, but hey…

'Tell me about it,' he said, his voice irritatingly gruff. 'We'll finish off and then you can go up to bed. I'll sit up with them and feed them.'

She cocked her head on one side. 'Does this happen often?'

That dragged a laugh out of him. 'Things rocking up at the door when we're shut? All the time—like you with Lola. If I had more cover, I'd still be running a night service, but I just haven't been able to recruit enough staff and when I do they leave because their partners have moved away with jobs or they're off on mat leave or they want a senior vet job—it just got relentless. So if this happens, it's all down to me to sort out.'

'Does everyone know you don't turn anything away?'

He grunted. 'Probably. I've no idea where she's come from, she was in a box by the gate. I expect someone got her on a whim and didn't follow through with a spay, and then didn't know what to do.'

'Is she microchipped?'

He shrugged wearily. 'I don't know. I haven't had time to check her yet. I'll do it when I've finished this, but I doubt I'll find anything. Let's get this done and get her settled and we can worry about it then.'

The little cat survived her ordeal, and so did all the kittens, but after a night spent taking it in turns to feed them, Ellie was drained.

So, by the look of him when he came down just before seven, was Hugo.

'You look about as good as I feel,' she said, and he gave a grunt of laughter.

'Don't. Coffee?'

'Please. Lots. And toast.'

'You do it, I'll check on the kitties and scan her for a microchip. And then I really need to take Rufus out for a run before we start.'

She looked at him a bit more closely and realised he was dressed in running gear. 'Really a run?'

'Really a run. We do it every day.'

'Wow. Where do you get your energy?'

His hollow laugh echoed in the empty air behind him as he went through to check on their little patients, and she went into the kitchen and realised she was smiling.

He was really getting under her skin...

The little cat had been microchipped, to his surprise, and she'd been reported as lost by her owners three months previously on the day they'd moved from Yoxburgh to Norfolk. Hugo rang them and they were delighted to hear she was OK, and came later that day. They left smiling with their little cat and her family, armed with cat food, kitten milk to supplement if necessary, and an advice leaflet.

'Nice to have a happy ending,' Hugo said to Jean after he'd waved them off.

'Nice to have your bill paid, even if it was heavily discounted,' she pointed out, and he laughed.

'Yeah, well, it wasn't their fault and I had to do it. Oh, and Ellie needs some overtime pay for that, too.'

'Overtime pay for what?' Ellie asked, walking into the office at the critical moment, and he left Jean to explain that to her. She'd only argue with him.

'What overtime pay?'

'For the cat. Her owners just came and collected them all. Didn't Hugo tell you?'

'No, I haven't seen him all day. So, what overtime pay?'

'Last night.'

'I don't need overtime pay for last night. And he needs to bill me for Lola.'

'Take it up with Hugo. I'm just doing as I'm told,' Jean said, and Ellie gave a little huff of irritation and went to find him.

'Why overtime?'

'Because you worked all night.'

'So did you. We did it for the kittens.'

'The owners came and got her and they paid the bill. It's covered.'

She tilted her head on one side and studied him. 'What, all of it, the whole, proper, everything-accounted-for bill? Or a figure you pulled out of the air because you felt sorry for them and the cat?'

'I'm not that magnanimous, but there may have been an element of that,' he admitted, but then trashed it by adding, 'and regardless of that, you still need paying for the overtime. And incidentally, while we're on the subject of magnanimous, you won't let me pay you locum rates, so you actually don't have a leg to stand on.'

'Fair cop,' she said with a chuckle, and walked away, but she hadn't forgotten that she owed him for Lola's treatment. She'd sort it out with Jean in a quiet moment, if there ever was such a thing…

CHAPTER FIVE

MERCIFULLY THE REST of the week was quieter—not that it was quiet, exactly, but certainly more manageable with the other two vets there on alternate days, and then it was Friday night.

To her relief she wasn't scheduled to work on Saturday morning, and she'd have time to spend with Lola at last.

She was still on cage rest, but she was well enough to move now. And Ellie really, really wanted to go to her house, even if it was only for the weekend. It would get them out of Hugo's hair and give her something else to think about apart from him.

She found him in the office at the computer, and she perched on the edge of the desk and waited for him to pause.

'Give me two seconds,' he said, and then pressed save and looked up with a smile. 'Sorry. You OK?'

'Yes, I'm fine. I'm going to my house tonight with Lola.'

He blinked. 'Really? I thought you were staying until she was off cage rest?'

'I know, but I'd like to be there, at least for the weekend, to give Lola a change of scenery if nothing else, and I need to get on with tackling it properly, as well. She can lie and watch me while I do stuff.'

'I'll give you a hand,' he said, without asking her if she needed help. Typical Hugo, and actually it was the last thing she needed when she was trying to get some distance between her and the man who was occupying all too much of her head space.

She shook her head. 'Don't worry, I can manage, but could I borrow your big crate for a while? Just until her stitches are out?'

'Sure, if you really feel you need to go, but you're welcome to stay here, you know that. The flat's just sitting there.'

'Yes, I know, but—'

'You want your own home,' he said softly, because of course, being Hugo, he understood.

She smiled. 'That sounds ungrateful, and I'm not, not after all you've done for me and Lola in the last week, but I thought if I spend the weekend there, I won't have to worry about her, I can get on with sorting my stuff out, and we can see how it goes. I'm assuming you won't mind if I bring Lola to work every day if I decide to stay there?'

'Of course I won't. She can lie in here in the day. She'll have plenty of company.'

'She will, and she was fine doing that at the other practice. If you don't mind, that would be brilliant.'

'Of course I don't mind. The crate probably won't fit in your car, but I can drop it over later, after I've taken Rufus out. Then I'll give you a hand, if you like?'

Did she like? She was torn, for all sorts of reasons. He'd done so much for her, and being independent was hard-wired into her DNA, but nevertheless it seemed churlish to refuse his help, like throwing his kindness back in his face.

'That's very kind of you, Hugo, but I can probably manage if you could drop the crate off,' she said, and hoped she could and it wasn't just a big fat optimistic lie…

Ellie pulled up on the drive with a feeling of déjà vu.

Was it really only a week since she'd arrived here so full of optimism and then everything had fallen apart? Just seven days, and without Hugo she had no idea what she would have done. Would Lola even have survived?

She felt her eyes prickling, and pulled herself together. No time for sentiment, she had things to do. She opened the front door and carried Lola in from the car and put her down, then looked around. She'd forgotten how tired it all was, how much in need of some love. She really needed to phone the agent and have a serious conversation.

She opened the back door and led her reluctant dog out into the garden. It was the first time Lola had been here since her accident, and she was a bit wary of it, but after a few moments of hesitation she was persuaded to step onto the grass—only for long enough to bop down and do a wee, and then she was back on the patio and staring pleadingly up at Ellie.

She clearly hadn't forgotten that the garden was full of terrors. Maybe tomorrow in full daylight would be better—under strict supervision, because even though Hugo had been meticulous, there might still be something lurking there and she'd never forgive herself if Lola was hurt again.

They went back inside, and Ellie took Lola's cone off. She wasn't allowed to jump up or go on the stairs until her sutures were out, so Ellie dug a throw out of the pile of bags still decorating the living room, spread it out in front of the sofa and sat down, patting the space beside her. Lola looked at the sofa, then at her, and lay down beside her with a sigh, head on Ellie's lap, and she fondled her ears.

'You're such a good girl,' she murmured, and Lola thumped her tail and sighed again. She could understand that. She'd be sighing all the time if she didn't stop herself.

'What am I going to do, Lola?' she asked, her voice weary. 'I wish I knew, but there's no hurry now, thanks to Hugo. Shall we see how it goes?' she asked the dog, and got another little tail thump in reply.

Not much of an answer, but heart-warming. Maybe it *could* be a home. And maybe Hugo really was as decent as he seemed. Should she take the job he'd offered?

Her chest tightened a little at the thought, and she shook her head. Too soon. There was no hurry, and besides, he still had to find a replacement, so she'd be locuming anyway for a while. She'd do as she'd promised and stick it out until then…

A car pulled up outside, and she heard the dull thunk of a door closing, then footsteps. She glanced out and saw him walking up her path, as if she'd conjured him up out of her imagination, and her heart gave a little skip. He was carrying a bag, and she opened the door as he rang the bell.

'Hi.'

'Hi.' He held the bag out to her, his mouth tipped in a crooked smile. 'I brought you something to eat. I wasn't sure if you'd had time to do a shop, so I dived into the supermarket.'

'Oh, Hugo, you didn't have to—thank you! That's so kind of you—or are you still trying to buy me?' she added, only half joking, and he gave a soft huff of laughter.

'You don't take anything at face value, do you?' he said, giving Lola a little tickle, and turned away and went back to his car.

Now she'd offended him—except he opened the boot, pulled out the crate, then leant in again and emerged carrying a plant in a pot. An orchid, the beautiful white flowers almost luminous in the dusk.

'What's that for?' she asked, expecting him to say yet another thank you for bailing him out, but he didn't.

His mouth tipped into another of those crooked smiles. 'Housewarming present. A little something to cheer the place up a bit—oh, and I've brought a body sleeve for Lola,' he said, and for a second she had the ridiculous urge to cry.

'Thank you, Hugo,' she murmured, absurdly moved by his simple but thoughtful gestures. She took the plant and beckoned him in.

'Sorry, it's still a mess. I haven't done a thing since I got here except sit down with Lola. Come on through.'

He followed her and Lola into the kitchen and put the shopping bag on the worktop. 'Does the microwave work?'

'I think so. I've cleaned it so I hope so.'

She put the orchid on the kitchen windowsill while he emptied the bag. Milk, eggs, bread, butter, tea, coffee, Greek yogurt, some fruit—and two ready meals.

'They're not exactly the healthiest, but I didn't think you'd want to start cooking on top of everything else. And I bought two, in case you fancied company?'

She searched his eyes, and all she found was that bone-deep kindness and consideration that seemed to be his trademark, and possibly her undoing.

'I don't have to stay,' he added, when she said nothing, and she swallowed another urge to cry—where was that coming from?—and found a smile from somewhere.

'Sorry. Yes, of course stay. What do I owe you for the shopping?'

'You don't give up, do you?' he said mildly.

'Not often.'

His lips twitched, and he pulled the receipt out of his pocket and glanced at it. 'Twelve pounds and seventy-four pence.'

She didn't believe him for an instant, but the receipt was back in his pocket and she tipped out her purse and found something close to it while he pricked the top of the ready meals and stuck them in the microwave.

While they heated she put the body sleeve on Lola and he erected the crate. He'd even brought a new sheet of thick vet fleece cut to fit it, something she hadn't even got round to thinking about.

She found a couple of plates that weren't too chipped, and they took their food into the sitting room and settled down on the sofa, Lola on the floor between them looking hopeful.

'Where's Rufus?' she asked, to break the yawning silence.

'In his bed. He's fine, he's had a busy day keeping an eye on things and he's had a bit of a run around in the garden, so I'll take him out later.'

The silence descended again, and she finished her meal—surprisingly delicious and very welcome—and then picked up their plates and took them back to the kitchen. He followed her and propped himself up against the worktop as she dumped them in the sink.

'Anything I can do? Carry stuff upstairs, shift furniture, help you make the bed?'

No way was he going anywhere near her bed, but the carrying…

'That would be great. I'll stick Lola in her crate while we do that, or she'll try and come up.'

'I'd put the cone back on, she'll need that unless she's under supervision,' Hugo said.

Lola wasn't impressed, but she went into the crate reluctantly and lay down with a great sigh, the plastic cone framing her mournful face.

'She does that martyr thing for England,' Ellie said with a chuckle, and led him back to the sitting room. 'Well, this is it. Grab a bag or two and follow me.'

She took the garment bag on top, followed by

a couple of carrier bags, and went up into her bedroom—*her bedroom? How odd*—and turned to find him right behind her with three bags in each hand.

'Where do you want them?'

'On the bed. That way I'll have to deal with them before I can go to sleep. Otherwise I won't get round to it.'

And it avoided the issue of him helping her to make it.

Except, of course, he had a better idea.

'Why don't we make it first, then dump the stuff on it? That way when you've finished emptying them you can fall straight into it.'

It made sense. Of course it did, so she searched the bags, found the bedding and quickly whipped out the mattress protector, the sheet and the pillow cases and dropped them on the mattress.

By the time she'd wrestled the duvet out of its bag he'd nearly done the sheet. In seconds the bed was made, and if it hadn't been for common sense she would have been tempted to fall straight into it there and then.

With him?

As they straightened up their eyes met, and she looked quickly away before he could see what she was thinking.

Madness. Tempted or not, there was no way she was going there. Not with Hugo, or any vet who was a prospective employer. Not after Craig, who'd made it impossible for her to stay in the job she'd only stayed in out of loyalty to Jim. And Hugo was a charmer. Her father had been a charmer, according to her mother, and she was never going to let herself fall for that.

But he was hoisting the bags back onto the bed, and she forced herself to meet his eyes again over the top of the heap.

'Coffee?' she asked lightly.

'Sure, if you've got time?'

'Of course I've got time.' And as he'd brought the coffee, it would have been churlish to kick him out without offering.

They ended up on the floor in the living room, Lola lying between them making the most of stereo cuddles, her head draped over Hugo's lap this time. The body sleeve had hind legs to cover the stitches, and she was groaning softly as he scratched her neck where the cone had been, and tugged her ears gently.

The movement of his hands was mesmerising, and Ellie looked away. She had to work with him, at least for the next few weeks or maybe months, and letting herself fantasise about his gentle, knowing hands on her body wasn't the way to do it. Especially with that freshly made bed right overhead…

Get a grip!

* * *

'So, what's your plan?' he asked, and she blinked at him.

'Plan?'

'For the house.'

She looked fleetingly relieved, for some reason, and he wondered if she'd thought he meant about the job. He already knew the answer to that, and it wasn't even as positive as a maybe.

'I don't really have one yet. Obviously it needs decorating from top to bottom, so I'll presumably start there, a room at a time, and then it'll need new carpets and furniture, really.'

'Especially if you're going to live in it for any length of time.'

She shot him a sideways glance and gave a wry smile. 'Nice thought, but I can't afford to replace anything yet.' She sighed. 'I need to phone the agent tomorrow morning. It's time I told him what it was like. And I still need to wipe down all the woodwork.'

'I can give you a hand tomorrow after we close if you like?' he offered without engaging his brain, and she glanced at him with that wry smile and looked away again.

'Hugo, I'm fine. I just need to put on my big-girl pants and get on with it.'

Why did she have to say that? He really, really didn't need to think about her pants...

'Well, the offer's there if you want to take

me up on it,' he said, and looked down at Lola. 'Sorry, sweetie, you need to let me get up, I have to go home and get on.'

'Admin again?'

He laughed, and it sounded hollow even to his ears. 'Always admin. Well, admin and Rufus. He needs a walk, or at the very least I need to play with him in the garden for a while. And I need to get that advert out there.'

He waited a heartbeat in case she picked it up, but she didn't, so he lifted Lola's head gently and slid out from underneath it.

'I'll see you out,' Ellie said, but he shook his head.

'You stay there with Lola. She looks comfortable. I'll let myself out. See you tomorrow?'

She tilted her head and smiled up at him, and he felt a jolt of something warm surge through him and settle in the region of his heart.

'You really don't need to help me. You've done enough already—more than enough. I can cope.'

'Big-girl pants,' he murmured, trying not to think about her bed right over their heads, and she smiled.

'Absolutely—and, Hugo?'

She reached up and caught his hand as he passed her, and the warmth turned to fire and burned through his body.

'Thank you. I don't know what I would have

done without you this last week. You've been a lifesaver. Literally, for Lola.'

He gave a little huff of laughter, and his smile felt crooked. 'I only did what you would have done, and as for Lola, that's what we do, isn't it? That's why we're here.'

He squeezed her hand, then disentangled his fingers and made his escape before he did something really, really foolish that would only hurt them both.

The front door closed with a firm click, and she rested her head back against the arm of the sofa and listened to the sound of his car driving away.

She could still feel the warmth of his hand in hers, still feel the unexpected quiver that had travelled through her like lightning, leaving longing in its wake.

No! No, no, no! She wasn't going to go there. Not that he'd suggested anything in any way, but…

'You're an idiot. He's just being nice.'

Lola lifted her head and stared at her, and she stroked her gently. 'Come on, baby, let's take you out in that beastly garden again and then put you to bed, hmm?'

She put their mugs in the dishwasher, then took Lola out, put the cone back on her and settled her in her crate before heading up to bed.

A strange bed, in a strange room, with all her

worldly goods piled on top of it, but she was too tired now to deal with that, so she dumped the bags on the floor, found her wash things and cleaned her teeth, then lay down on the unfamiliar mattress, staring at the ceiling.

Her own bedroom, in her own home.

It should have felt wonderful, but it didn't, it felt oddly wrong, temporary, uncertain. There was still so much that was undecided, so many ways to go, different paths to travel.

Should she take the job? Or just locum for now and take the time to do up the house a bit and then re-let it and move on? But where to? She'd have to find accommodation that would take Lola, and that was tricky. And she couldn't take her with her into practices if she was locuming, it wouldn't be fair on any of them.

Only one thing was certain. If she stayed here, she'd definitely need a better bed…

She spent Saturday morning washing the woodwork downstairs with Lola, but she needed to pull out the washing machine and dishwasher so she could clean under them.

Except that meant asking Hugo for *another* favour.

'Oh, Lola, what am I thinking? I need to leave him alone! He's got a life, and he doesn't need us clogging it up.'

Lola lifted her head and thumped her tail gently on the floor. Thank goodness she'd got her. She'd go mad otherwise.

And she'd still be in her old practice working with the odious Craig.

'It's a lovely day, let's go and have a look in the garden, shall we?'

She managed to drag and lift the crate out onto the patio, and Lola went hastily into it the moment she opened the door. She left it open, so Lola could come out if she wanted to, and then spent an hour or more peering down into the grass to see if she could find anything else that might present a hazard.

Not easy, as it needed another cut already and of course the lawnmower in the little shed was useless, the cable sliced through as if it had been mown by accident.

By the time she was satisfied that it was safe, Lola had come out of her crate and was lying on the patio in the sun watching her, so she sat down beside her, a hand on her side, and stared blankly at the garden.

If you could even call it that. Another thing on her endless to-do list.

She took Lola inside, hauled the crate back in—harder than bringing it out, of course—and put her back into it, then went into town. First stop the rental agent, only the office was closed, so she found a supermarket, bought a few food essentials, a pot of violas in full bloom to cheer up the garden, a packet of drawer liners and some dishwasher and washing machine cleaner, then headed back.

The first thing she did was run the empty dishwasher and the washing machine on a hot wash with the cleaner, then spent an hour adding to her to-do list and emailing the letting agent, then went for a short stroll while Lola was napping, trying to find some nice walks for her once she was able to start controlled exercise again.

She did the same thing the next day, heading towards the sea this time, and of course she bumped into Hugo and Rufus out on a run.

He slowed to a halt and stopped in front of her, his chest heaving, sweat dribbling down his neck and into the running vest that clung to his lean, toned frame, and her heart lurched in her chest.

How is it that, even hot and sweaty, he's so darned sexy?

'Hi,' he said, his eyes crinkling into a smile, and she smiled back and bent to say hello to Rufus. Not that Rufus really cared, but it was a good excuse and got her eyes off his body.

Except his legs were now right in front of her, and they were every bit as distracting as the rest.

'You look hot,' she said, and then could have kicked herself, but he just laughed.

'I am hot. I'm steaming. We've just done ten K, ready for the race next weekend.'

'Race?'

'Yes, there's one every year in aid of the local children's hospice. I've been tapping the clients for sponsorship.' His grin was cheeky and made her heart hiccup, and she had to look away again. 'So how's it going?'

'Oh, OK. I'm just taking a little stroll to keep my muscles working and to get to know the area ready for taking Lola out,' she told him, distracting her brain from the subject of his hot sweatiness and his support for charity, both of which made him even more attractive than he had been.

Why does he have to be so nice?

'How's she doing?'

'OK, but she's bored to death. I reckon in another week her leg should be healed enough so she can come out of prison. She'll love that.'

'She will. It's nine days now.'

'Yes, I suppose it is.' Ten since her world had been turned upside down, and nine since she'd met him—

He shifted from foot to foot. 'I'd better go or I'll stiffen up, I need a shower and some stretches, but what are you doing later?'

How to find an excuse to avoid him? 'Trying to tame the house?' she said truthfully, and then without permission her mouth tacked on, 'Why?'

He shrugged. 'I thought, as the weather seems so much warmer today, I could crack out the barbecue? Then Rufus and Lola can spend a bit of time together and it'll give her a change of scenery. She must have serious cabin fever.'

She wasn't alone, just the thought of tackling the house made Ellie want to run away, and the offer was so tempting. Still, she really shouldn't…

'That sounds lovely. Anything I can bring?' her mouth asked, and she contemplated sewing it shut.

'No, nothing. I've got some stuff in the freezer and I'm going shopping after I've showered. Two-thirty?'

She nodded, cross with herself for being weak and yet looking forward to it because she felt oddly lonely here. Lovely though everyone here was, she missed her friends in the old practice, and her house with all that needed doing was overwhelming. And a barbecue with Hugo…

'Two-thirty's fine. Are you sure I can't bring anything?'

'Just yourselves,' he said, and she told herself that the invitation was as much about Lola as it was about her. If not more so.

'OK. I'll see you then.'

He threw her a smile and set off again, Rufus running beside him, and she watched him go, those long, strong legs eating up the pavement, and kicked herself for being so weak-willed.

Maybe she should start applying for other jobs.

And leave him in the lurch, after all his kindness?

No. She couldn't. And she knew in her heart of hearts that she ought to put him out of his misery and take the job, but she was scared of doing it, scared of making another mistake, another wrong decision, another error of judgement—

'He's nothing like Craig,' she told herself crossly as she walked back into the house, and Lola looked up at her and whined. She opened the crate and stroked her head.

'I'm sorry, sweetie, you have to stay in there. You need a rest before this afternoon, and I need to get *something* done on the house. Maybe it's time to fire up the washing machine. What do you think?'

It didn't really matter what Lola thought about that as an idea, because the washing machine needed another hot cleaner wash before she'd want to use it, and anyway, she didn't have time to dry the clothes before tomorrow. She phoned Hugo.

'Can I ask a favour? Can I use the practice washing machine? I'm running out of clothes.'

'Of course you can. Bring everything over when you come. In fact why don't you just come back today instead of tomorrow? It would save moving Lola backwards and forwards and you won't have to rush in the morning.'

She hesitated, torn between her need for distance from him and the lure of the blissfully comfortable bed in the flat.

The flat won hands down, and she didn't really want the distance, anyway, if she was honest. 'Thanks, you're a star. I'll do that.'

She hung up, had a shower, threw all her washing into a bag and then rummaged through her clothes.

'It's not a date!' she told herself crossly, and threw on a pair of jeans and a top, then changed the top for a nicer one, grabbed a jumper just in case it got chilly later, and then loaded Lola and the laundry into the car and headed back to the practice.

He'd opened the gate for her, and she shut it behind herself and parked in her usual place, then picked Lola up and carried her round to the staff entrance. She could see Hugo in the office, and she put Lola gently on the floor and took her in there so she could say hello.

'Are we interrupting?'

He gave a wry, tired laugh and reached out to give Lola a little love. 'Not really. I'm posting an ad for the vet job. I thought I'd throw in the flat, see if it tempts a few applicants.' He tilted his head to one side. 'Since I clearly can't tempt you?'

Oh, she was so tempted, but there was no way he was knowing that…

'What?' he asked, his brows crunching together, his eyes searching. 'Are you having second thoughts?'

She looked away. 'I'm not sure. Right now I'm not sure about anything.'

He gave a grunt of laughter. 'Well, if it helps give you a little certainty, how about I take you on as maternity cover for Lucy, then that gives you time to decide and me time to find a permanent replacement if you really don't want to stay?'

'When's she due back?'

'Six months, give or take.'

Six months…

She held his eyes for a moment, then looked away again. 'Can I think about it?'

'Sure. Of course you can. And I'll hold fire on the advert for now.' He pressed save, closed his laptop and got to his feet. 'Let's go and cook. I'm starving.'

'Can I put my washing on first?'

'Help yourself. I'll get started, come on out when you're done. I'll take Lola with me, I can tie her to the bench and she can lie in the sun and hang out with Rufus.'

CHAPTER SIX

BY THE TIME she'd put the first load into the washing machine there was a delicious waft of barbecue in the air.

She went out into the garden and found Hugo, armed with tongs, standing by the barbecue with the contented look of a man making fire, Rufus and Lola gazing up at him hopefully.

'It really smells of summer out here,' she said, and he turned his head and grinned.

'About time. It's been cold too long. I've got a very attentive audience.'

'Yes, I can see that,' she said with a smile. 'Lola's leg certainly hasn't affected her appetite.'

'Have you had a look at it today?'

'Yes. It's healing beautifully, thanks to you.' She peered at the laden griddle. 'That looks delicious. Anything I can do?'

'Yes, you can relax.'

Relax? It was so long since she'd truly relaxed she wasn't sure how to do it, but she parked herself on a sun lounger, lay back and closed her eyes and let the sounds of the garden wash over her.

She could hear the hiss and spit of the barbecue, the scrape of the tongs as he turned things on the griddle. A bird was singing somewhere in the garden, and she could hear another answering it. Blackbirds? Maybe.

The sun was warm on her skin, not the fierce heat of summer, but the gentle warmth of spring that relaxed her muscles, emptied her mind of her worries and lured her into sleep…

It was ready. Hugo turned the barbecue down, piled all the food on the warming rack and closed the lid.

He turned, his mouth open to speak, and then stopped.

'Ellie?' His voice was low, no more than a murmur, but she didn't respond, and his mouth softened into a rueful smile. He didn't have the heart to wake her.

Her chest was rising and falling slowly, her limbs relaxed, and he made himself look away. He really didn't need to know what she looked like when she was asleep, her face unguarded, her body motionless apart from the gentle lift of her breasts towards the sun with every slow breath…

God, he wanted her. He wanted her so much it hurt, but she deserved so much more than he could offer.

He closed his eyes, but he could still see her, see the soft curves, the peep of cleavage in the vee of her top—

Should he wake her? She clearly needed to sleep.

He opened his eyes and saw a wasp on her cheek. Her eyelids flickered as her hand came up to swat it away.

'Don't move, it's a wasp,' he said quietly. 'Just keep still and it'll go.'

It flew off, and she sat up and turned towards him, looking a little confused, her eyes blinking against the sun.

'Sorry, I must have dropped off. How long have I been asleep?'

He shrugged. 'I don't know, I've been busy. Five minutes, max? I was about to wake you when the wasp landed. The food's ready when you are. I'll bring out the salads.'

Had he been watching her sleep?

Idiot, of course he hadn't. She was reading far too much into it. Why would he want to watch her anyway?

He came back out with a tray and set it down on the table, and her smile felt awkward. 'I'm sorry, I didn't mean to drop off like that, but it was just so relaxing in the sun.'

'You obviously needed it.'

She nodded. 'Yes, I guess I did. I didn't sleep well last night.' Or the night before…

He paused in mid-unwrapping of the salads and turned to look at her searchingly. 'Why?'

She shrugged. 'I don't know. Maybe the bed? It's not because I'm not tired, but—I don't really know. I just feel so unsettled.' Partly because of him, but there was no way she was telling him that—

'I'm sure you do. There's been a lot of sudden change in your life and it must have been pretty overwhelming. I know how that feels, but you've got a job here for as long as you want it, and a very decent reference if you want to move on, so you don't need to worry about that.'

Except she did, because somehow it all seemed too cosy. And it wasn't that she couldn't trust Hugo professionally, that was a given, but she felt this weird pull towards him, an almost visceral yearning, and it was herself she didn't trust. She was in danger of falling in love with him, and that wasn't in any way a good idea. Not personally, not professionally, and certainly not now.

'I know,' she said, breaking away from that searching gaze, 'and I am very grateful for all of that, but it's everything else as well,' she said, making excuses now. 'There's so much to do on the house, and I don't know where or how to begin. I need to speak to the letting agent, really.

I've emailed him asking for a meeting. I might need to take some time off for that, if it's OK?'

'Sure.'

'Not that it'll make any difference. He'll probably just say it was "wear and tear", knowing my luck.'

Hugo grunted and picked up the tongs. 'Very likely. Right, we're good to go. Grab a plate and come and load it up.'

They ate in silence, the dogs lined up watching every mouthful while he watched Ellie.

She looked troubled, and after what she'd said, he wasn't surprised. He could offer to help with the decorating, but he really didn't have time while they were so short-staffed. And if he offered to pay a decorator, she'd only say no.

'Do you want this last sausage?'

She shook her head, so he put the leftover salads in the fridge for lunch tomorrow and shared the sausage between Rufus and Lola.

It was starting to cool down now, the sun dropping lower in the sky, and despite her thin jumper he saw her shiver.

'Coffee?' he suggested, and she gave a tiny shrug.

'I feel so guilty. I really ought to be at home getting on with something,' she said. 'My to-do list is ridiculous.'

And she didn't sound as if she wanted to do any of it.

'It'll keep. Come on, let's go and get a coffee. It'll be warmer inside and we can talk through what needs doing before you speak to the agent.'

She hesitated, a host of emotions flickering in her eyes, and then she nodded. 'That sounds good. You're right, the house can wait.'

She had a message from the agent just before eight the next morning, suggesting he meet her at the house. Now.

She stared at her phone, sighed and went to find Hugo.

He was in the office with Kerry, running over the list of consults and electives while Jean answered the phone and slotted in another client.

'Hugo, I'm so sorry to do this, but is there any way I can meet the agent at my house now? He's just messaged me.'

He hesitated for a second, holding her eyes, then shrugged. 'Sure. We can cope.'

'Thanks. I've fed Lola and she's been out, so she should be fine. I'll be as quick as I can,' she promised, and headed off armed with a list of issues and very few expectations. It was going to be a difficult meeting and it needed to be done, but she was so not looking forward to it…

While Jean went out to Reception, he and Kerry rejigged the first couple of appointments. Difficult, as he didn't know how long she'd be. Would she get any joy from the agent? He doubted it, and he certainly wasn't holding his breath—

'Hugo? Hello?'

He shook his head to break his train of thought, and looked back at Kerry. 'Yeah. Sorry. What?'

'Is Ellie OK?'

'Yes, she's fine, she's just got issues with her house. The tenants pretty much trashed it.'

'Mmm, she said that the other day. It sounds a nightmare.'

'It is a nightmare, and it all needs decorating, which is difficult when she's living in it.'

Kerry pounced on that immediately.

'Let her stay on in the flat as long as she's here. You aren't going to find a new vet that quickly, not anyone worth having, anyway. They'll have to give notice. And it's just sitting there doing nothing. It's the obvious solution.'

It was, and he'd already thought about it.

'It would give you a chance to get to know her better, too,' Kerry went on, and he searched her eyes and turned away, letting out a frustrated huff of laughter.

'Don't start that. I don't need you matchmaking.'

'But she's lovely, Hugo, and you're lonely—'

'I'm not lonely, I don't have time to be lonely, and I'm hardly a monk.'

'I'm not talking about your sex life, Hugo, I'm

talking about a meaningful relationship. You've been on hold for ten years—'

His heart crashed against his ribs. 'You don't have to tell me that, I'm well aware,' he said shortly.

'Don't you think it's time—'

He glared at her. 'Don't go there, Kerry. I'm warning you…'

'She'd be so perfect for you.'

She would be. She was. She wasn't the problem, he was. Not that he was telling Kerry that. 'Just because you're all loved-up—'

'That doesn't mean you can't be. James and I don't have the monopoly. You deserve to be happy.'

He shoved a hand through his hair. 'Dammit, do I have to fire you to get you to shut up?' he growled, his pent-up frustration threatening to boil over, but she'd known him a long time and she just smiled gently and shook her head.

'Have it your way, Hugo, but you know I'm right. I just want you to be happy,' she added over her shoulder as a parting shot, and he waited till she'd gone and punched the wall.

Hard.

He rubbed his knuckles, the pain bringing him to his senses. Kerry was right. Ellie was perfect for him, in every way. But he was very far from being perfect for her, and the past kept coming back to haunt him.

He clenched his fist again, but it was already sore enough so he left the wall alone before he broke a metacarpal and went and called in his first client.

The flat idea was still kicking around in his brain, though. He'd initially offered it to Ellie as the obvious solution while Lola was on cage rest, but she was almost better now, and Ellie still hadn't committed to cover Lucy's mat leave.

Even though he knew letting her stay on in the flat for longer was the ideal solution for her, it would put them in very close proximity for however long it took to fix her house, which would do nothing to help keep any distance between them.

Except she needed to get the house sorted, and that would give her a chance. And then there was his other idea that would help her even more—although it would throw them together for even longer, so that was still kicking around in the back of his mind.

He was such a sucker for punishment…

Ellie headed back to the practice, still not quite believing how the meeting had turned out, and Kerry grabbed her on the way in.

'How did you get on with the agent?'

'He's agreed to refund his commission, which means I can afford to get it decorated. I can't believe it.'

Kerry blinked. 'Wow. That's a result.'

'Isn't it?' She just hoped Hugo wouldn't mind

her staying on in the flat a bit longer, but then Kerry pre-empted that.

'You won't be able to live in it while that's happening, of course,' she said, ever practical, 'but Hugo won't mind if you stay on in the flat. It's sitting there doing nothing.'

'At the moment, but he's going to offer it to a new vet so he won't want me there for long.'

'You're covering Lucy's mat leave, aren't you?'

'Well—only for now. I haven't agreed to stay—'

'Well, that's fine, he can still advertise the job with the flat. The decorating won't take long, will it?'

It wouldn't, once she'd found someone to do it, but…

Then Kerry moved on. 'Anyway, enough of that, I've been meaning to ask you if you'd like to come to my wedding in three weeks? The day's for family, but the evening's a party and I'd love you to be there. Everyone here's coming, and you're one of us now.'

Was she? Was she really 'one of them'?

She waited for that familiar feeling of the net tightening, like it had in her last practice whenever Craig had organised social events for them and she'd felt obliged to go, but it didn't happen, because this wasn't Craig, it was Hugo. His practice, his head nurse. All she felt was the steady, gentle warmth of welcome, and she felt her eyes fill with unexpected tears.

'Oh, Kerry, that's so sweet of you. I'd love—'

Kerry beamed. 'Great. I'll add you to the list. You can be Hugo's plus one.'

She stared at Kerry. 'Hugo's…? But surely he's got someone to bring? A girlfriend?' she added, now blatantly fishing, but Kerry just shook her head.

'Hugo? No, or certainly not one he'd bring to the wedding. He doesn't have time.'

Didn't he? Or was he just lonely, and filling time with busy work? What a waste of his life—and actually, none of her business.

'Kerry's invited me to her wedding,' she told him later between consults, and he gave a wry smile.

'I didn't think it would take her long.'

Really?

'So how did you get on with the letting agent?' he asked, changing the subject swiftly.

Ellie shook her head slowly and laughed. 'Weird. He was a bit defensive, but then acutely embarrassed when he looked through my photos, said he'd sent a new member of the team out to deal with it and should have done it himself. And, amazingly, he's refunding me all the commission from the last six months, which means I can afford to get it decorated.'

She let it hang, wondering how to bring up the

flat, not wanting to put him in a difficult situation because knowing Hugo he'd just say yes regardless of his own feelings.

'That's great news. Look, I don't have time to talk now, I've got a Lab with an obstruction, but let's get this morning out of the way, and we can talk over lunch. I've got an idea I want to put to you.'

'Is this the mat leave thing?'

'No. Later.'

Except that lunch didn't happen for either of them, not surprisingly, and it was after six before her last client left. She walked out of Reception and bumped into him in the corridor.

'Sorry about lunch,' he said, 'the Lab took longer than I thought.'

'What was it?'

He rolled his eyes. 'Foam balls from the park. He'd eaten at least two, judging by the colours, and his gut was choked with bits, some of them huge. I don't know why people give them to dogs. They get chopped up when they mow the grass and some dogs just can't resist. Have you got time now to talk?'

'Sure, I'm not busy. I just need to eat pretty soon, so as long as it doesn't take more than a few minutes I'm fine, otherwise we can do it after I've eaten. And I need to spend time with Lola.'

He laughed. 'It'll take seconds. Let's do it now,

and then I'll cook us something while we talk about it.'

'It's not your turn,' she pointed out, but he just laughed and headed upstairs anyway.

She left Lola in the kennel and followed him up, curious. His door was open, so she walked in and propped herself against the worktop in his kitchen while he pulled stuff out of the fridge.

'What have you done to your hand?' she asked, eyeing a nasty bruise on his knuckles.

'Oh, nothing, I misjudged a doorway,' he said, sounding a bit short, and carried on sorting through the fridge.

'So what did you want to talk about?' she asked as he straightened up.

'The flat.' He had his back to her as he chopped veg, so she couldn't read his expression, but his shoulders seemed a bit tense. 'I know what it's like trying to work on a property and live in it, and it's not easy, but if you're going to get a decorator, it'd be much easier for you and for him if you'd moved out, and the flat's the obvious answer.'

'Kerry said I should ask you about doing that, but I thought you might not want me in it for that long,' she said carefully.

He glanced at her then looked away again, turning his attention back to the onion he was dicing into a million pieces. 'Why wouldn't I want you in it?'

Why wouldn't he look at her?

'I don't know. Because you want it for the permanent vet, when you get one? Because I'll be in your way?' she tacked on, wondering if that was it, but he shook his head.

'You won't be in my way.'

'But it's not necessary. I don't have to move out, Hugo, I can just stay there and they can work round me.'

'You don't need to do that, not when the flat's just sitting here, and anyway, I'd already assumed you'd be here. That's not really what I wanted to talk to you about,' he said, scraping the onion into the pan before turning to face her and coming up with something that took her completely by surprise.

'I've been thinking. If you cover the rest of Lucy's mat leave, which is six months, that takes us to mid-October. If you move into the flat and stay here all summer, rent free, which is the vet's deal, then you could get the house done up a bit and rent it as a holiday let. They're in very short supply at the moment, and Yoxburgh's really popular in the summer.'

She stared at him, vaguely stunned because it had never occurred to her, and it was a genius idea. Except…

'I know. We used to holiday here when I was a kid, and I loved it, which is why I bought the house, but that isn't the point. What if you find a really good vet who's available sooner and they need accommodation? I'd have nowhere to go.'

He shrugged. 'Then let your house as a late last-minute deal. If you want to, of course. I just thought it might help pay the mortgage.'

She stared at him, stunned.

It would. It absolutely would, and the money would be really useful, because having lost nearly three months' rent due to the tenant, she didn't have much of a buffer, even with the commission being refunded. But…

'Can I think about it?'

'Sure. I'm doing Thai paneer curry. Red or green?'

She stared at him blankly for a second, then gave a soft laugh. 'Green would be lovely. Thank you. Let me go and feed Lola and take her out for a minute, and I'll be with you.'

By the time she'd done that he was dishing up, to her relief, and they sat at the table and ate without speaking until their plates were cleared.

Then he pushed his plate away and looked up, his head cocked on one side as he met her eyes. 'So, has the agent suggested a decorator?'

Ellie swallowed the last delicious mouthful and shook her head. 'No, and I wouldn't know where to start looking.'

'I spoke to Ryan, the guy I use, while you were downstairs with Lola. He's got a gap next week if you're interested. I said I'd call him back if you were.'

Another thing to be beholden to him for? He'd picked up their plates and headed over to the dishwasher with them. Was it her, or was he really avoiding her eyes?

'Is he expensive?'

'Yes and no, because he's quick, so he doesn't waste time and he's very, very good, and he clears up after himself. He used to do work for Peter, and he's done quite a bit for me. Or you can find someone else? Up to you.'

'How is he available, if he's any good?' she asked sceptically.

He shrugged. 'People pull out for all sorts of reasons. Financial pressure, mostly.'

She stared at his back, knowing that it made sense, debating the 'beholden' thing again, since they were talking about financial pressure. But if he was a known quantity…

She gave up. 'OK. If you give me his number I'll call him.'

'I'll do it, I said I'd come back to him.'

Which probably meant he'd offered him some financial incentive, she thought, knowing Hugo, but he handed her his phone after a few brief words, and two minutes later she had a decorator lined up, an appointment to meet him at the house tomorrow evening at six thirty, and a promise that he could start on Monday.

She gave Hugo his phone back and chewed the inside of her cheek.

'What?' he asked, studying her with those eyes that saw altogether too much and right now gave away too little.

'Nothing. It just seems too easy—'

'That again? Life doesn't have to be difficult, Ellie, and you can trust Ryan. Yogurt and berries?'

'On one condition. I'm cooking tomorrow, as soon as I get back from the house.'

He held her eyes, and one corner of his mouth twitched. 'You're on. Do you want some colour charts to look at? I've got some somewhere.'

The decorator was bang on time, and she was back in the practice by seven. Hugo, predictably, was in the office, Lola and Rufus at his feet, and he turned to her as she went in, his eyes searching her face.

'How did you get on?'

'Quite well, I think,' she said, giving Lola a love. 'He said he could get it all done next week. He's sending me a quote this evening. It'll probably be hideous.'

'Great. I've done my run, so are you cooking, or am I ordering a takeaway?'

'I'm cooking. Give me ten minutes.'

The quote pinged into her phone while she was cooking. It made her wince a little, but the house would be transformed in a few days and she could move on with her life. If nothing else, she'd have options, and Hugo's suggestion of letting it over the summer was growing more tempting by the minute.

She showed the email to Hugo when he appeared. 'What do you think? Is that fair?'

He nodded thoughtfully and handed her phone back. 'I would say so. It's about what I expected, maybe a bit less. I'd bite his hand off. What colour are you going for on the walls?'

'White everywhere except the front door, because it's cheaper and easy to touch up. I'm just worried it'll look too clinical.'

'No. It'll look clean and fresh, especially if you're going to let it?'

She searched his eyes. 'Are you really OK with that? Because it seems a brilliant idea—short term, only, obviously, and no longer than Lucy's mat leave, but it would give me a buffer.'

'Of course I'm OK with it. I wouldn't have suggested it if I wasn't.' He leant over and peered into the pan she was stirring. 'That smells good. I'm starving. Anything I can do?'

She emailed Ryan and accepted his quote, and then the next two days were so busy she didn't have time to worry about her house. Hugo's charity ten K was coming up on Sunday and he went running every evening after work, sometimes for half an hour, sometimes for longer, and she took the time to take Lola out into the garden and let her wander around for a good while before going inside to cook for both of them.

He argued, of course, but she pointed out she owed him, and if nothing else it was good for her pride.

'Chosen a colour for the front door yet?' he asked on Thursday while she was cooking, and she shook her head.

'I have no idea.'

So after they'd eaten they went down to his flat and he dug out the colour charts and they sat together on his sofa poring over the coloured squares and drinking coffee.

'That's nice,' he said, pointing to a very dark blue. 'Sort of charcoal navy. It could look very smart.'

She peered at the colour he'd picked out, leaning closer and catching a delicious whiff of shampoo and warm skin. She straightened up, her own skin warming, her heart rate kicking up a notch.

Why? Really, why? I need to get out of here...

She shifted away. 'Yes, I think that one could look great. Can I hang on to the chart and show it to Ryan?'

'Of course. Or drop him a text. He'll pick it up then before he starts. More coffee?'

'Uh, no, thanks, I've got stuff to do, and I want

to take Lola out for a little stroll. I think she's healed enough now and she must be so bored.'

'I'm sure she is. That's fine. I'll see you in the morning.'

He listened to the door close, and dropped his head back and blew his breath out slowly. Why on earth had he suggested she should do this? It was bad enough bumping into her during the day, but the evenings, eating together, sitting together over coffee, chatting about this and that, it was all too cosy, too—dammit, too tempting.

That worried him. There was no way this was going anywhere, however tempted he was. He wasn't in the market for anything other than a decent vet to cover Lucy's mat leave. Nothing more, and certainly nothing like what his body was screaming at him to do. He saved that for women who didn't expect anything from him but a good time. And now he and Ellie would be living cheek by jowl for months.

This was all Kerry's fault.

No, it isn't. You brought it on yourself.

He flexed his fist, but it was still sore, so he left the wall alone…

Ellie ran upstairs, closed the door of her flat and leant back against it. Why was she reacting like this to him? She'd known him two weeks now—two weeks tomorrow. She worked with him, ate with him, and mostly it was fine, but then every now and again he'd be that little bit closer, close enough to smell the scent of his skin, feel the warmth radiating from his body, and her heart would somersault in her chest and she'd feel breathless until he moved away.

It was ridiculous. And if she was going to be living here over the summer, letting her house, she was going to have to get a grip. And maybe a bit more space. Fewer cosy evenings…

That was fine. She could do that. Lola was almost better now, so every evening she could take her for a walk, a nice slow stroll onto the clifftop to look at the sea, then a stroll back via the other road. Starting now.

She put on her trainers, ran back downstairs and let Lola out of her kennel. 'Come on, sweetie, I've got a lovely treat for you. We're going for walkies.'

Lola's ears pricked, and she seemed more than ready to go out. They wouldn't be long, Ellie wouldn't do that to her on her first proper outing, but she needed to build her strength and have a change of scenery, and so did Ellie.

Especially scenery that didn't have Hugo in it…

The sun was setting as they reached the clifftop, and she watched the light on the water, the slow, lazy swell of the waves washing away the stress. The tide had reached its height, she guessed, and she sat on the grass, Lola lying down by her side, and they watched the sky turn a glorious orange streaked with purple while all the tension faded away.

Lola nudged her with her nose, and she gave her a hug and got to her feet. 'Come on, little lady, let's take you home.'

And hopefully Hugo wouldn't be in the office…

Sunday dawned cool and sunny, with a light breeze, to Hugo's relief.

The run kicked off at ten, and he was mercilessly collecting last-minute sponsorship from anyone he could.

He'd already tapped the practice team, and Ellie had chipped in with twenty pounds that he knew she couldn't afford until she was on a better footing, but he'd taken it anyway.

He couldn't see her here today. Maybe she was at the house getting it ready for Ryan to start tomorrow, or maybe she just didn't want to come, but as he scanned the crowd he saw Peter and Sally waving as they made their way towards him.

Bless them, they never failed to support this event, and he knew they'd sponsor him generously. They always did.

'Hugo,' Peter said, wrapping him in a hug and

slapping his back fondly. 'How are you? Ready for this?'

'I reckon. I've been putting in some pretty good times.'

'I'm sure you have,' Sally said, kissing his cheek and hugging him. 'Where's your form?'

He handed it to her, and over her shoulder he caught sight of Ellie. He beckoned her over. 'Ellie, I'd like you to meet Peter and Sally. Ellie's the vet covering Lucy's maternity leave.'

'Good to meet you, Ellie, I've heard great things about you,' Peter said, shaking her hand warmly.

'Good to meet you, too, and I've heard wonderful things about you both. It's nice to put faces to the names.' Her smile seemed warm and genuine to Hugo's eyes as she shook their hands, but he noticed she didn't really look at him. Well, not in the eye, at least—

No! He didn't need to think about her now, he needed to focus on the run and remember why he was doing it. Not that he could ever forget… 'Right, guys, I'm going to shoot off and warm up. I'll see you when it's over.'

'We'll be here,' Sally told him, and handed back the form.

He glanced at it. 'That's ridiculously generous.'

'It's not for you,' she pointed out, and he hugged her hard and headed for the group gathered behind the start line, his heart pumping.

* * *

As he jogged away, leaving Rufus with Peter, Ellie's shoulders dropped a notch, as did her heart rate, and yet again she wondered what on earth she'd committed herself to by agreeing to locum until October—never mind living in the flat!

Sally smiled at her, but her eyes were assessing and Ellie wondered what his godmother was thinking. Peter, thankfully, had better things to do making friends with Lola.

'This must be the invalid we heard about,' he said, rubbing her tummy and studying the faint line of the scar on the inside of her thigh.

'Yes—well, she was. She's not now, she's pretty much healed, but Hugo was—amazing. Not that I gave him much choice, I pretty much bullied him into treating her, but without him I don't know what would have happened to either of us.'

Peter gave Lola a last pat and straightened up. 'No, he told us a little about it and I don't think you had to bully him. He's a good lad. Always has been. Priorities in the right place, but he—he's had a lot to deal with.'

She met his eyes and read a warning there, a gentle reminder that Hugo, too, had been damaged and needed care.

'I know, he told me. He also told me how wonderful you both are, and how much love and support you've given him. And judging by you being here today, I guess you still do.'

'We do. Right, I think we need to head over there, Sally. We can catch up later, Ellie. I think we're all going to the pub.'

He and Rufus walked away, heading after Hugo, but Sally hung back.

'Peter's right, we do try to support him however we can, but there are some things we can't fix,' she said, her eyes following Peter as he walked towards Hugo at the race start point then looking back at her as she added softly, a gentle warning in her eyes, 'Please don't hurt him.'

Ellie shook her head. 'I—I'm just working there. We're not...'

'He said you've become a friend.'

'Did he?' That warmed her in a way she hadn't expected. 'Yes—yes, I suppose I have, in a way, but—that's all it is. We're not...'

'That's a shame,' Sally said softly under her breath, and followed Peter to the start line, leaving Ellie staring after her, not knowing what to make of that.

'Hey, Ellie, come on, we have to watch them set off,' Kerry said, linking her arm through Ellie's and towing her and Lola towards the start.

She went, a little reluctantly, Sally's words echoing in her head. 'Please don't hurt him.'

And what about me?

CHAPTER SEVEN

THEY WATCHED THEM set off, Hugo at the front of the pack, and as the runners streamed past them, Kerry turned to her.

'Right, let's go and find a coffee and a doughnut and have a look round the stalls. There are all sorts of things—puzzles, books, clothing, local produce, tombola, splat the rat, a bouncy castle for the kids, and it's all in aid of the hospice so I hope you've brought lots of money?'

'I brought some,' she said, wishing now that she'd brought more cash because she'd had no idea there'd be so many stalls. 'How long have we got?'

'Before the front runners get back? About forty-five minutes.'

'And Hugo?' she asked, wondering if that sounded too needy, but Kerry just chuckled.

'Hugo won it the year before last, but last year someone pipped him, so he'll be right up there trying to get that title back.'

'Is that why he's been training so hard?'

'Oh, no, he always pushes himself. He's a bit driven, really, but it's not surprising. He's had so much to deal with.'

'Yes, he told me. It was awful.'

'He told you?' Kerry glanced at her, her face surprised.

'Yes. We had a long heart-to-heart,' Ellie said softly, remembering their conversations about his parents, and his mother dying in a hospice would explain his support for this one.

Kerry sighed. 'I'm so glad he felt he could open up about it. They took such wonderful care of them all for the short time he was in there.'

He? Ellie stopped in her tracks. 'He?'

She stared at Kerry blankly, and Kerry stared just as blankly back, then let out a long groan.

'He didn't tell you, did he? Oh, no…'

'Tell me what?'

Kerry closed her eyes and bit her lips. 'Oh, Ellie. I should have realised he wouldn't have told you. He never talks about it.'

'About *what,* Kerry? What does he never talk about? I know he lost both his parents. I thought you must mean his mother dying in a hospice?'

Kerry shook her head, and Ellie could see she was fighting back tears. She felt a cold chill spread through her.

'Who is "he", Kerry?' she asked, dreading the answer.

She hesitated, then said softly, 'His baby.'

His baby? His...son?

'No...'

'Don't say anything to him, please? I shouldn't have told you, and it'll only upset him.'

She shook her head. 'No, no, of course I won't. I...'

'Come on, let's go and get a coffee and sit down for a bit,' Kerry said, and steered her towards a picnic bench by a refreshments stand.

'So—what happened? Where is he now?' she asked, half of her not wanting to hear the answer, but Kerry's face was enough. 'He died. Didn't he?'

Kerry nodded wordlessly, and Ellie felt the air sucked out of her lungs. Her eyes filled with tears and she blinked them away, but they slid down her cheeks and she swiped them away. 'I had no idea,' she said, heartbroken for him. 'How—that's...'

'Sorry. Look, I'll get us a coffee. Stay here.'

Stay? She couldn't have moved if she'd tried. She sat down on the bench as if her strings were cut, staring numbly across the field while Lola sat pressed against her leg. To comfort her?

She could see runners in the distance through a gap in the hedge, streaming past. Was Hugo at the front, driven by the need to support the place that must mean so much to him? Or just running away from it, trying to forget...

No. He'd never forget. You couldn't. But how

could he live with that? Live with such a horrendous, soul-destroying loss? It must have torn his heart out…

She closed her eyes, the tears leaking through her lids and streaming down her face, and she felt something pushed into her hand. A paper napkin, offered to her by Kerry who was sitting beside her with a coffee in her hand and a bag of doughnuts on her lap.

She scrubbed her face, blew her nose and sniffed hard. 'Sorry. It just—'

'I know. And I'm the one who's sorry, I didn't mean to dump that on you. I shouldn't have—'

'When?' she asked, her voice sounding weird and somehow remote. 'When did he die?'

'Nearly ten years ago? I'd just started there. It was before Peter retired, and Hugo dropped off the face of the earth for a lot of the time in those few months. How he would have coped without Peter and Sally I don't know, and of course it was the nearest they'd get to a grandchild, so they felt the loss almost as deeply. And he hasn't had a meaningful relationship since. It broke him, and I think he's scared of the what-ifs.'

'What what-ifs?'

'In case it happens again—maybe. I don't know. He just shuts down if you raise the subject. He'll talk about anything else, but not that.'

That made sense. 'He told me about himself, about his parents dying—and actually, when he was telling me that, I was sure there was something else. There was just some undercurrent, and he suddenly changed the subject and asked me about myself. It was right back at the beginning—I hardly knew him at all, and we told each other all sorts of stuff, but not that. Never, ever that—'

She pressed a hand to her mouth to hold in a sob, and Kerry put an arm round her shoulders and hugged her.

'I should have realised he wouldn't. I don't think anyone else at the practice knows apart from Jean who's been there for ever, and she never gossips. Here, have a doughnut. They're still warm, and you probably need that sugar hit.'

She took one, the sugary crunch followed by soft, sweet dough and the comforting squelch of jam. She took another bite, and another and another, almost absently, then handed the last bit to Lola, dusting off her fingers and dredging up a smile.

'Thanks. You were right, I needed that.'

'You're welcome. Come on, let's drink our coffee and have a wander round before we go back and wait for them. We've got twenty minutes or so.'

They stood at the finish with Peter and Sally and other members of the team. While she was still trying to make sense of what she'd been told, they were yelling and cheering as he ran through the timer beam, then slowed and ducked under the tape to join them. He bent over, hands on his knees, chest heaving, his body driven to the limit, slowly getting his breath back.

Then he straightened up and checked with the stewards, and came back to them with a broad smile.

'Ten seconds off my PB,' he said, but the smile didn't quite reach his eyes—not now she knew what to look for.

'Congratulations,' she said, and then turned and slipped quietly away, the tears threatening again as she left him, surrounded by the nearest thing he had to family.

Ten years of sorrow, ten years of loss, ten years of denying himself a family, the children he'd be such a good, kind, loving father to.

Don't hurt him.

We're just friends.

That's a shame.

She walked quickly away, taking a reluctant Lola with her, and a moment later she felt a firm, warm hand on her shoulder.

'Hey, where are you going? I thought we were all going to the pub?'

She couldn't look at him, not now, with those tears still threatening, not knowing what she knew.

'Sorry, I need to get on with the house. Ryan's

coming in the morning and I need to get it ready. But well done. I'm really pleased for you.'

She glanced up fleetingly then and caught the flicker of a frown on his face as she forced a smile. 'I'll see you tomorrow.'

'OK,' he said, the words coming after the briefest hesitation. 'Shout if I can help.'

'I'll be fine,' she told him, her voice much firmer now, but her smile was probably no more convincing, so she turned and walked away, taking a still reluctant Lola with her.

Hugo watched her go, torn between the people behind him and the woman in front.

Something was wrong, he had no idea what, but she didn't want to talk to him. Sure, there must be things she had to do at the house, but he didn't think sorting the house was enough to make her cry. And she'd been crying, without a shadow of a doubt. Why?

He turned and walked slowly back to the others, endured a stream of hugs and back-slapping and handshakes as the results revealed that he'd won, and then he caught Kerry looking at him with an odd expression on her face.

He moved to her side. 'What's up with Ellie? Why's she crying?'

She shook her head slowly, biting her lip. 'We need to talk.'

'Well, go on, then, spit it out.'

She closed her eyes and shook her head again. 'It's my fault, Hugo, I'm so sorry. She was asking why winning was so important to you, and I said you always push yourself hard. I said you were a bit driven, you'd had a lot to deal with, and she said she knew, you'd told her, and I just assumed…'

'You told her.' He crushed it down, the rush of emotion he thought he'd outrun, but he hadn't. He never could.

'Not in so many words, but you seem to be so close—'

'Not that close.'

Never that close, not to anyone, never again…

'I just said the hospice had been very supportive while he was in there, and she just stared at me. She thought I was talking about your mum, and after that I had to tell her—had to explain. I'm so sorry, Hugo, you know I would never have told her if I hadn't thought she knew.'

Her eyes were welling up, and he sighed and gave her a quick hug. 'It's OK, it doesn't matter, it's done now. I'll talk to her later. Right now I need a shower, and then we're going to the pub to celebrate.'

'Really?'

'Yes, really. We don't have a choice. Chin up, Kerry, what's done is done and it's not the end of the world.'

* * *

She heard a knock at the door in mid-afternoon, and she froze.

Hugo? Who else? Anyone else, hopefully, because if it was Hugo she wouldn't know how to look him in the eye.

She peered out of the window, but there was no car outside. Not that that meant anything, he was quite likely to have walked. Or it could be one of the neighbours come for a nose round. Please God…

Except Lola was whining and scratching at the door. The knock came again, and she braced herself and opened it.

He was standing there with Rufus, hands rammed in his jeans pockets, unsmiling, and she could see the pulse beating at the base of his throat.

'Hugo, I said I didn't need your help.'

'I know.'

She closed her eyes, not sure what to say, not sure what to do, but he took the decision out of her hands.

'Can we go for a walk?'

She looked at him again, her heart pounding, but his eyes were blank, giving nothing away. Not so the tension in his body. Had Kerry told him?

'Yes, of course. I'll put Lola in her crate.'

They walked side by side in an awkward silence, Rufus sniffing along the way, and when they reached the cliff top they made their way down the steps and along the concrete walkway, the sea stretching away to their right, the water glinting in the sunlight.

She didn't say anything, she had no idea what to say or where to start, so she left it up to him. A couple passed them, going the other way, and still she waited. And then finally they reached a point where the concrete ran out and the rocky sea defences took over, and at last he stopped walking.

'I spoke to Kerry.'

What was she supposed to say to that? She had no idea, so she said nothing, and he carried on.

'I asked what was wrong with you. She said—' He sucked in a breath, then let it out in a shaky rush. 'She said she'd told you about Samuel. Thought you knew.'

Samuel. She hadn't known his name, and somehow knowing it made her hurt for him even more.

She closed her eyes, and the tears slid silently down her cheeks. She felt him brush them away with a gentle hand.

'Hey, come on. Let's sit down.'

They sat side by side on the shingle, shoulders not quite touching, Rufus wedged between them.

He laid a hand on the dog's head, stroking it gently, and then he started to speak, his voice low, sombre.

'We weren't married—we'd been on and off for a bit and we weren't together any more, and it was a while before Emma realised she was pregnant. She had a scan at twenty weeks which showed that the baby had all sorts of issues and he might not even survive the pregnancy. She contacted me then to tell me about it, so even though we weren't together, I was there for her. I had to be. He was my child as much as hers, and I blamed myself for her getting pregnant. She didn't want a termination, she wanted to let nature take its course, and he was born at thirty-seven weeks.

'His DNA had three copies of chromosome eighteen in each cell, instead of the usual two. It's called Edwards' syndrome, or trisomy 18, and the fault could have come from either of us. They said it wasn't a heritable defect, just one of those things, a failure in the cell division of the ovum or sperm, but in his case it was incompatible with life.

'His head was small, and he had cysts in his brain, which meant sometimes he stopped breathing, and he had difficulty swallowing so he had to be tube-fed. His heart wasn't plumbed right so his circulation was impaired, so he was on oxygen, but he wasn't in pain and he wasn't in imminent danger of dying and he didn't need to be in the noisy hospital, so we got him moved to the hospice so we could be with him in a quieter, more normal environment for as long as he had.

'And they were wonderful in there. He needed round the clock care, so with their support we took it in shifts, and then when he was eight weeks old he got a chest infection, and he died in my arms—'

His voice cracked, and she rested her head against his shoulder, her hand on his arm.

'I'm so sorry, Hugo.'

His hand covered hers. 'Don't be. He couldn't have lived, his body was too compromised, but that time we had with him was so precious. It'll be with me for ever, but I couldn't go through all that again.'

'What about Emma? She must have been devastated.'

'Oh, she was, of course, but she's moved on. She's married now, she's had three children. I don't know how she could do that. It would seem all wrong to me, somehow, to have another child, as if I'd airbrushed him away because he didn't matter. But he did—'

His voice cracked again, and he stopped talking, the tension vibrating through him, and a single tear leaked out of the corner of his eye.

Oh, Hugo...

She closed her eyes, and he put an arm around her and leant his head against hers as they sat in silence, listening to the sound of the sea lapping on the shingle, each lost in their thoughts.

And then he straightened up, sucked in a breath and gave her a crooked little smile. 'We need to go and get your house sorted out.'

He stood up, held out his hand and pulled her to her feet, then wrapped his arms around her, folding her against his body as if to comfort her, and as he spoke she could feel the low rumble of his voice.

'Don't be sad for me, Ellie. I'm OK.'

Was he? Was he really? She didn't think so, not for a second.

She kissed his cheek, and he turned his head and his mouth brushed hers and lingered for a moment, then he lifted his head, leaving her lips bereft and her body aching to comfort his.

She laid her head against his chest, felt the slow, heavy thud of his heart against her ear, and after the longest moment she straightened up and moved out of his arms, but he didn't let her go, just slid his hand down her arm and took hold of her hand and held it all the way back to her house while she thought of his baby and tried not to cry.

She unlocked the door and went in, and he followed her and the silence closed around them, still unbroken, the tension now replaced by sorrow.

'I don't have any dust sheets,' she said inconsequentially, dragging them both back into the here and now, and his mouth twitched into a smile that didn't quite reach his eyes.

'Ryan has hundreds of dust sheets. Let's get your stuff out, give him a clear field.'

An hour later her possessions were stacked in her bedroom at the practice.

All except the beautiful orchid he'd given her, and she'd put that on the worktop in the kitchen so she could see it every day.

'Have you eaten?' he asked, and she shook her head.

'You have, though, haven't you? You went to the pub.'

His smile was a little twisted. 'I didn't eat a lot. How about we try again, just the two of us and the dogs?'

So he took her to the Harbour Inn, and they had fish and chips and shared some with the dogs, and gradually she began to relax again.

He drove them home—funny how the practice and not her house seemed like home—they went upstairs together and he kissed her, another gentle touch of his lips on hers that left her heart and her body aching.

'Goodnight, Ellie,' he said after a breath-stealing pause, and turned away.

She nearly called him back, but that would have been foolish, and anyway she needed some time alone to think. She heard the door on the landing click shut, and she closed her eyes.

'Goodnight, my love,' she whispered, and closed the door, walked into her bedroom, lay down on the bed and cried for him.

* * *

Within days the house was transformed.

So was her relationship with Hugo.

She felt she had a much greater understanding of him, and she could absolutely understand Sally's 'don't hurt him'. Her 'that's a shame' was echoed in her heart, but there was no way he was going to take their relationship any further, so they focussed on the friendship that they'd formed.

With the run over for another year, their evenings were spent walking the dogs, often strolling along the beach or beside the river. Sometimes they'd eat out, sometimes she'd cook for them, sometimes he would.

And as soon as Ryan was finished, she got her house ready for holiday letting, found a site where she could advertise it and within moments she had her first tenants lined up.

'Wow, that was quick,' he said when she told him.

'It was. I'm stunned. I just hope they don't trash it. And of course it's taken my eye off the ball for this wedding and I don't even know if I've got anything to wear. What's the dress code? And do you have any idea what I could buy for them?'

'Black tie, and no. She's got a gift list on a website, I believe. Ask her.'

'I will. And I might have to go dress shopping.

I've only got three days and I've got to get the house ready, they come on Sunday.'

'That's fine, you can do that whenever. There are some good shops in Yoxburgh, nice little independents and they aren't outrageous.'

They didn't need to be outrageous, because she didn't have money to fling around after the expense of the house. She asked some of the others what they were wearing, and they were all going in long. And she didn't have a long dress.

Unless she wore the wrap dress she'd got for Jim's retirement party…

It was hanging in her bedroom in the flat, and at lunchtime she ran up and pulled it out. Would it do? She'd felt good in it, she'd only worn it once, it had been expensive, and it was long.

Well, it was at the back, but not at the front where it wrapped across. That was mid-calf.

Long enough? Probably. And it was a beautiful dress.

She stripped off her scrubs, put it on, tied the waist and looked in the mirror, but it wasn't a full-length mirror so it was hard to judge. A bit too much cleavage? And if it was windy…

But she owned it, it suited her, and it picked up the colour of her eyes.

'It'll be fine,' she told herself, and hung it back up.

Job done. Now she just had to buy a present.

* * *

Hugo gave his bow tie a last little tug to straighten it, looked at himself in the mirror and closed his eyes.

He really, really needed to find a smile or he'd upset everyone, but he wasn't looking forward to the wedding.

It would have been easier without Ellie being his 'plus one' as Kerry, so blatantly matchmaking, had described it. They'd grown closer since the race, and he was finding it difficult enough to keep his distance as it was, especially since he'd kissed her. OK, it had been pretty platonic, but that had only been because he'd firmly kept it that way.

If she'd been anyone else, they would have ended up in bed weeks ago, but she wasn't a woman he could sleep with and kiss goodbye, and that was as much of a commitment he'd been prepared to make for years. And he cared about her far too much to want to treat her like that.

But with all the romantic wedding vibes, the alcohol, the dancing—hell, especially the dancing.

His heart sank. He'd be expected to dance with Ellie. They'd all be watching and waiting for it, and he'd bet his life that as soon as they were up on the dance floor Kerry would get the DJ to play some slow numbers, and she'd end up in his arms.

No alcohol, then. The only thing left for him

to influence. Unless she hated dancing. He could only hope—

There was a quiet tap on the door, and he opened it to find Ellie there, looking drop-dead gorgeous in a beautiful dress that did absolutely nothing for his increasingly fragile self-control. It was bad enough when she was wearing scrubs—

'Will I be all right in this?' she asked doubtfully.

If it was any more all right he'd die of a heart attack, but that was his business, not hers. He dragged his eyes off the soft swell of her breasts so perfectly framed by the vee.

'Yes, it's fine,' he said, his voice gruffer that usual because that dress had totally emptied his brain. 'It's lovely. Are you ready?'

'Yes, I'm good to go.'

She needn't have worried about her dress. It was just right for the tone of the occasion, and she felt good in it.

They'd left the dogs together in his flat and walked to the venue, arriving bang on time, and after she'd changed into heels and left her wrap and flats in the cloakroom, they'd gone in and found some of the others from the practice there clustered around the bar talking to Kerry and her new husband James.

'Oh, she looks gorgeous,' Ellie said softly, 'and so happy, both of them.'

'They are, and she deserves it. I'm really happy for her.'

Kerry turned then and spotted them, and after all the kisses and hugs and handshakes were done and they moved on, Hugo turned to her.

'What would you like to drink?' he asked her, and she hesitated, then threw caution to the winds.

'White wine? Just a small one, not massive, I'm a bit of a lightweight and I haven't eaten yet.'

'No, nor have I. We'll have to raid the buffet later.'

He ordered drinks for all the practice members there, got himself an alcohol-free beer, handed her the wine and they mingled with the others.

'Hello, you,' a voice said behind them, and Hugo turned and gave the woman a warm hug.

'Lucy! Great to see you, I'm so glad you're here. Lucy, this is Ellie, she's covering your mat leave.'

Ellie met her eyes—curious, assessing—and smiled at her. 'Hi.'

'Hi. I've heard a lot about you from everyone. I hope Hugo's not working you too hard.'

She laughed, wondering what she'd heard, hoping none of it was idle speculation. 'Not as hard as he works himself, that's for sure. And everyone's been lovely.'

'They are lovely. I miss them.'

'I hope that means you're coming back,' Hugo said, and Lucy laughed.

'Never say never,' she said, 'although I might pop in soon.'

'Do. You're always welcome. So, how's it going?'

'Great. I love being a mum. Sleep would be nice, but—yeah, it's all good. Anyway, I need to mingle, we're not here for long and I've got loads of catching up to do. See you soon?'

'Sure.'

Lucy turned away and went back to the others, and Ellie met Hugo's eyes and smiled. 'She's nice.'

'She is. Right, somewhere there's a buffet table, and I need to eat. I had half a sandwich for lunch.'

They grazed on the buffet, mingled a bit more, and then it was time for the first dance.

They all clustered round to watch, phones clicking as photos were taken, videos filmed, and then everyone clapped and cheered and headed onto the dance floor.

Hugo looked down at her with a smile she couldn't quite read. 'Shall we?' he said, and held out his hand.

She put hers in it, and a shiver of something strange ran up her arm and settled in her chest, robbing her of breath. She should have had a bigger glass of wine, she thought, and let him lead her onto the dance floor.

The music was typical wedding dance stuff, and despite his apparent reluctance, he was a natural. It didn't surprise her, because he always moved fluidly, but it was years since she'd danced with anyone who didn't have two left feet, and it was a joy to dance with someone who loved it as much as she did.

And then the music slowed, and he held out his arms and she moved into them. Not too close, but close enough that she could smell the subtle fragrance of his cologne, feel the light touch of his hand on her back, the occasional nudge of his legs against hers, and her body caught fire.

She glanced at his face and met his eyes, and with a quiet sigh he eased her closer; she rested her head on his shoulder, his cheek against hers, his body close now, his legs brushing hers as they swayed together to the music. She felt his lips graze her cheek, and she turned her head a fraction and his mouth met hers, a light, fleeting kiss that seared all the way down through her body, leaving her feeling more alive than she had for years.

He swore softly, then turned his head a fraction, his mouth by her ear, his voice a low murmur.

'We need to get out of here.'

They did, but she had no idea where it would lead, and she had no more idea where she wanted it to lead, either.

She just knew that for now, she wanted Hugo, and he wanted her, as simple and as complicated as that.

Except there was nothing simple about leaving, because Kerry caught them on the way out and gave them both a knowing look.

'Damn,' he said after they'd made the feeble excuse of needing to get back to the dogs and headed for the foyer.

'Don't worry, she's had way too much to drink, she probably won't even remember,' Ellie said, hoping it was true.

She retrieved her ballet flats, slung her wrap around her shoulders and they walked back to the practice, not quite touching, not quite apart.

So what now?

What was he doing? What was he *thinking* about?

He had no idea, he just knew that the only sure way to find out where this was going was to go with it, and go with it they would, he knew that much.

Either that or he'd die wondering what it would be like to—

He put his key in the lock, let them in and led her up to his flat.

The dogs gave them a rapturous welcome, and he took them out into the garden for a moment and came back up, wondering if she'd still be there or if she would have come to her senses and gone up to her flat.

No such luck.

'Stay and have a drink?' he suggested, leaving her a way out, just in case, hoping to God she didn't—

'Sure.'

She didn't look sure, and he wasn't, either, but it made no difference. He headed to the kitchen. 'Coffee or wine? I have both.'

'What are you having?'

Second thoughts, but he didn't say that, because she turned and he caught a flash of leg where the two sides of the dress met, and his brain left the building.

He swallowed. 'I don't really want a drink,' he said, and held her eyes.

Then what...?

'Nor do I.'

He held out his hand, and she let him draw her into his arms.

'I want you.' His voice was gruff, and she could feel the tension vibrating through his body. It matched the tension in her own, and she lifted her head and met his eyes.

'I want you, too,' she whispered, and he closed his eyes.

His mouth found hers, tentatively at first, then bolder, his teeth nipping lightly at her lips, his tongue teasing, coaxing, and then hot, so hot as she opened her mouth to him.

He rocked against her, his erection hard against her abdomen, one leg nudging between hers as he lifted her against him, his mouth doing incredible things to hers.

And then he broke away and let her go.

'I think we need to take this somewhere—'

'Horizontal?' she offered, and he gave a strangled laugh.

'I was going to say without the dogs, but yeah, that too.'

He shut the dogs in the sitting room, then caught her hand in his and led her into his bedroom and closed the door.

'So, where were we?'

'Not horizontal yet,' she said with a shaky smile, and tugged at his bow tie. 'Oh. It's real.'

'Of course it's real.' He slid it out from under the collar and laid it on his chair, shrugged off his jacket, heeled off his shoes and turned back to her. Then he stopped, took her by the hands and stared down into her eyes.

'This isn't going anywhere, you know that, don't you?'

She nodded, not at all sure if that was how she felt but willing to go along with it. So long as he was…

'If you don't want this, I can go,' she said, but

he shook his head and his mouth tilted into a wry smile.

'Oh, I want. Believe me, I want.'

He cupped her face in his hands and kissed her again, slowly and thoroughly, then let her go and took a step back. 'We have way too much on,' he said, his voice hoarse, gravelly with need, his eyes so dark they looked almost black.

He turned off the top light, put on a bedside light and stripped off his shirt—or tried to. 'Stupid cufflinks,' he muttered, and she took his hands and slipped the cufflinks out one by one, dropping them on his bedside table.

When she turned back his shirt was gone, and his hand was on his belt buckle. She stopped him, removed his hands, undid the buckle, slipped the leather free, then reached for the waistband. Two clips. Why so many?

And then his zip was sliding down, and she let go and his trousers slid down his legs and puddled round his ankles.

She closed her eyes then, unable to look at him without touching. She heard the soft rustle of fabric, a muted clunk as the belt buckle hit the floor again, then his hands were on her waist.

'How does this undo?'

She reached for the bow and he caught her hands and eased them aside, then she felt the waist fall away, the cool air of his bedroom brushing her skin as he opened the front of the dress.

She heard the sharp hiss of indrawn breath, felt the touch of his hands on her shoulders brushing the dress aside so it slid to the floor, then his hands reached around her and unclipped her bra and freed her aching breasts.

She opened her eyes and they locked with his as he reached for her and drew her into his arms, his chest heaving as if he'd been running, the soft hairs chafing lightly at her nipples with every breath.

His kiss was long and slow, one leg nudging between hers, the thin layers of fabric between them annoying now.

'Hugo, please,' she said, her voice cracking, and he tugged back the covers, stripped off his shorts and then slowly, inch by inch, he drew that last tiny scrap of lace away, his mouth following it.

She sucked in her breath, and he straightened up, lifted her and laid her on the bed, following her down and straddling her. Then he reached into the bedside table and pulled out a small foil packet, tore it open and took out a condom.

'I'm on the pill,' she told him, but he just shook his head.

'I still want this.'

'Let me,' she said, and, in the gentle light that gilded his body, she saw the muscles in his abdomen clench as she touched him, carrying out the intimate task with deliberate and meticulous care. He tipped his head back and swore softly as she trailed her trembling fingers slowly back up.

He took her hand away. 'Are you done torturing me?' he said, his voice uneven, his breathing ragged.

She couldn't stop the smile. 'I think so. For now.'

He stared down at her, his mouth tipping into an answering smile, and then the smile faded as his hands reached down and cupped her breasts, taking his sweet time as he rolled her nipples gently between thumb and forefinger, then shifted down her body, bending his head to draw her nipples one at a time into his hot, hungry mouth.

His tongue toyed with them, his teeth nipping gently, his lips closing over them as he suckled. She bucked and writhed under him, and finally, when she thought she was going to cry with frustration, he nudged her legs apart and slid slowly, deeply inside her.

A long, shuddering groan echoed through his body and into hers, then his mouth found hers in a kiss that nearly sent her over the brink as he began to move. His hands were everywhere, nothing off limits, and so were hers. She loved the feel of his body, the taut muscles of his shoulders, the feel of his hair sifting through her fingers, the slight roughness of his beard against her cheek as his tongue flicked against the pulse in her neck. The tension she could feel building in him…

She was close, so close, and then he shifted again, his clever, knowing fingers touching her, coaxing her, taking her over the edge and then following her with a guttural cry as his body stiffened against hers.

He lowered his head and rested it against hers, and she could feel his breath hot against her shoulder.

And then, as the echoes faded and their breathing slowed, he rolled away from her, got up and went into his bathroom, closing the door behind him with a soft but definite click.

CHAPTER EIGHT

HUGO DEALT WITH the condom, then propped his hands on the washbasin and stared at himself in the mirror, shaken to the core.

What the hell just happened?

Apart from the fact that he'd just had the most profound sex of his life. He closed his eyes and groaned.

Why? Why the hell did you do that?

No idea. No idea at all, except it had seemed like a good idea at the time, get rid of the urge, take the edge off it. But it hadn't, had it? No. It was worse than ever, because now he *knew*. He knew just how good it was with her, and it scared him, because sure, the sex had been good, but it had been more than that.

Far more.

He felt like he'd given her his soul, and taken hers. So now what did he do with it? Hand it back? Tell her it was all a stupid, rash mistake and they should never have done it?

He had no idea. He just knew he wanted her

like he'd never wanted anyone ever before and, whatever happened, it was going to hurt them both.

She tugged the covers over herself and lay there motionless, staring at his bathroom door, her body still thrumming with the last echoes of her climax.

So what happens now? Is that it? Is he done with me now?

No idea. Should she get up and leave before he told her to go? Get up and put her dress back on and go and sit with the dogs? She could hear them whining in the other room, wondering what was going on.

They weren't alone.

The bathroom door opened and he walked out, gloriously, beautifully naked, and she wanted to touch him, to hold him, to make love with him again. But she didn't have the right to do that, because it would make it more than just a one-off drunken quickie.

Not that it had felt like that, at least for her. Quick, yes, but something much more powerful, more meaningful than she'd expected. And neither of them were drunk, or at least not on alcohol, so that meant—what, exactly?

'The dogs are whining, and I'm still hungry. Fancy a snack and a cup of tea?'

He turned away before she could read his eyes,

and she stared at his back. He was lifting a bathrobe off the back of the door, shrugging into it, covering that glorious, wonderful body that had just taken her to places she'd never been before and stolen her heart along the way.

'Sure,' she said, although she wasn't sure of anything right then. 'I'll run upstairs and put something on.' Something sensible that didn't give out such blatant signals…

'I'll be in the kitchen.'

He left the room, and she scrambled out of bed, flung her dress back on, scooped up her underwear and shoes and ran up to her flat, closing the door behind her and leaning back on it with a shaky sigh.

She had no idea what was going on in his head, and his eyes had been unreadable. Mostly because he'd had his back to her for nearly all of that very brief conversation…

She hung up her dress, pulled on fresh underwear and her jersey PJs, and then after a glance in the mirror she took off her makeup and went back down to his flat, her heart beating a tattoo behind her ribs.

He'd pulled on sweat pants and a hoodie, and he was busy in the kitchen, the dogs at his feet looking hopeful.

'That smells good,' she offered, trying to sound normal.

'I made cheese on toast,' he said over his shoulder. 'Hope that's OK.'

And he turned then and smiled at her, and she still couldn't read his face, but at least he wasn't frowning. He picked up the laden plate.

'Here, you take the tea and I'll bring this. I don't want Rufus to steal it, he loves cheese.'

'He'd have to fight Lola for it,' she said drily, and smiled back, not sure if it would look like a smile or some kind of weird rictus, but it was the best she could do. She picked up the mugs and followed him.

Rufus and Lola, as predicted, were all about the cheese, dancing around under Hugo's feet, their eyes fixed on the plate.

'No. Lie down.'

They lay, obeying him but eyeing the plate longingly as Hugo sat down beside her with it on his lap.

'Here, let's eat it quick while it's still hot and before they drool everywhere.'

She took a slice, the melted cheese running off the edges of the toast, stretching into strings as she lifted it. She scooped it up, wiped it off on the crust and sucked the tip of her finger, then glanced at Hugo.

He was watching her, transfixed, and she could read his face easily now. Want, need, the white heat of that visceral urge that had brought them together just a short while ago.

'Did you have to do that?' he said, his smile wry, his voice not quite managing to be casual.

'I'm sorry—'

'Don't apologise,' he told her, and leant over and kissed her. Just a touch, a light brush of his mouth on hers, the flick of his tongue to catch the taste of that melted cheese.

Then he leant back, his shoulder against hers, and picked up a slice, biting into it with a groan that dragged her mind straight back to his bed. 'Oh, that's *so-o-o* good! I'm starving.'

She couldn't watch him. Too tempting, too—just too *Hugo*…

His arm settled round her shoulders, pulling her in against his side as he rested his head against hers.

'Are we OK, Ellie?'

His voice was low, a little gruff, and she turned her head a fraction so she could see him, the food forgotten.

'I don't know,' she told him frankly. 'Are we?'

His mouth twisted a little. 'I hope so. But I think we need to talk.'

She looked down at her cheese, cooling now, congealing on the toast as it cooled. 'Can we eat and talk at the same time?'

She felt as much as heard his chuckle.

'Yes, we can eat and talk.'

But he didn't talk, so she prompted him.

'So what did you want to say?'

He'd just taken another bite, so he shook his head and chewed and swallowed, a smile playing on his lips. She was happy to see the smile, because she had no idea what was coming and until he got on with whatever it was he wanted to say—

'Sorry. OK. Firstly, I have absolutely no regrets about what happened. But if we're going to do it again, we need some ground rules first,' he added, his smile fading.

Ground rules? 'OK,' she said slowly. 'Such as?'

He hesitated, his smile well and truly gone, his face serious now. 'I don't do permanent. I don't do long-term, I don't make promises I can't keep—and I don't want anyone else here knowing. And there's no way you're getting pregnant if I have anything to do with it.'

The last one was clearly a veiled reference to Samuel, and maybe all the rest of his rules, too. She chewed and swallowed, taking her time while she tried to work out exactly what he was saying. 'So, is that it?'

He turned his head and studied her face for a moment. 'I think so, for now. Your turn,' he added, but she shook her head.

'I haven't—I didn't ask for permanent, I didn't ask for long-term—'

'You didn't ask me to leave the wedding with you so abruptly and come back here and—'

He broke off, and she wondered, for a moment, what he'd been going to say.

'Make love to me?' she suggested, her words hanging in the silence, and he met her eyes again, his utterly unreadable this time.

'I don't do love,' he said.

Because love hurt, she realised, and he'd already lost too much. Oh, Hugo…

She felt something in her chest squeeze a little tighter. 'OK, so what do you do?' she asked, and then added bluntly, 'Apart from having mind-blowing, earth-shaking no-strings sex?'

She'd felt it, too?

The blown mind, the shaken earth.

The soul-sharing? She hadn't mentioned that. Maybe she hadn't felt it the way he had.

'That's pretty much it,' he said, his voice a little terse because he wanted to deny it and couldn't. He wasn't going to talk about the soul-sharing, not now, not ever. He had nothing to offer her. Nothing that would expose him to any more losses in his life. His heart was like a hollow shell already. Letting himself fall for her would just tear out the little that was left of it when she went. Which she would, in the end. And she deserved better than the little he had to offer.

'OK.'

He stared at her, his mind distracted. 'OK?'

'Yes. OK. Your terms.'

He pulled himself together. 'And what are yours?'

Something raw and hurt flickered in her eyes and was gone before he was sure.

'I don't do Ts & Cs, Hugo, and I'm on the pill and you're using condoms, so that takes care of that one. All I'd ask is that you don't slag me off to all the practice staff when you decide you're done with me.'

He swore, dumped the plate and turned her face towards him, appalled. 'I would never do that to you. *Ever.* And the last thing I want to do is hurt you.'

He leant in and kissed her, just a fleeting, gentle touch, an apology for sounding like a—

'No!'

He swore again, snatched up the empty plate and glared at the dogs. They were gulping down the last few pieces, and they didn't even have the grace to look guilty…

'Come back to bed,' he said, and then added, as a belated afterthought, 'Please?'

She couldn't have said no to him if her life had depended on it.

They took it slower this time, savouring every touch, every tremor, every kiss, and when it was over he kissed her gently, rolled away and went into the bathroom.

She watched him go, wondering what would happen now, what his protocol was for this kind of event. Would he expect her to go up to her room for the rest of the night? Stay here with him? And what about the dogs? Lola was used to being upstairs with her now. Where would *she* sleep?

Maybe she should just be proactive and get up—

The bathroom light clicked off, and he walked back to the bed, turning off the bedside light as he got back under the covers. 'Come here,' he said softly.

He rolled towards her, drawing her into his arms again, and his kiss was tender. 'You OK?'

'Mm-hm. You?'

'I'm very OK.'

He kissed her again, then rolled onto his back, leaving his arm around her, and she lay with her arm draped over his chest and her head on his shoulder, listening to the beat of his heart and the slow rhythm of his breathing.

I don't do love.

Maybe not, but he did mind-blowing, earth-shaking no-strings sex with bells on. Maybe she should have said heart stealing, too. Because that was what it was. She felt as if he'd reached inside her chest and cradled her heart in his hands, and nothing would ever feel the same again, and she wanted to cry…

He woke in the night to raging thirst and a dead arm.

She was fast asleep, her body lax, her breathing slow and regular. He eased his arm out from under her, tucking the pillow in its place, and went quietly out of the room, snagging his robe off the back of the door and wincing as the blood flowed through his arm again.

The dogs were silent, so he left them alone and went into the kitchen, downed a glass of water and then made a cup of tea and sat and drank it, his mind lost in thought.

Was she really OK? Would they be able to do this? He didn't know, and the very last thing he wanted to do was hurt her, hurt anyone, but she was young, only early thirties, and she had so much life to live, so much love to give.

It would be so easy to let himself love her, but she deserved a family, not a no-strings contract, and that was all he could offer her. All he *dared* to offer her. And it wasn't enough.

Idiot. You shouldn't have touched her.

He swore softly under his breath, and stared blankly out of the window. The sky was still dark, not even the slightest touch of pale along the horizon, but he was too wired to sleep. He scrolled through the photos he'd taken last night, Kerry dancing with James, a group one of the practice members, and then one of Ellie laughing at him that got him right in the solar plexus.

And then just because why not torture himself, he scrolled back through the photos, right back to ten years ago and his photos of Samuel.

There was one of him lying in Emma's arms, another in his own, one of his little finger in Samuel's tiny fist, another with Peter and Sally.

Four broken hearts, four lives plunged into grief and despair. A salutary reminder of why it could never happen again…

He switched off his phone, put it on charge and went quietly back into the bedroom. She was motionless, silent, and he let his robe drop to the floor and lay down, easing the duvet over himself.

'Are you OK?'

Her voice was soft, concerned, her hand finding his shoulder in the darkness, and he shifted to face her. 'I'm fine,' he lied. 'I was just thirsty.'

'You've been ages.'

'I made tea. We didn't drink the last one.'

'I know. I'm thirsty, too. What's the time?'

'Three twenty-eight the last time I looked. Want me to get you tea?'

'Tea would be lovely. Thank you.'

He made them both one, and took them back to the bedroom. She'd turned on the bedside light and she was in the bathroom, and she came out naked and beautiful and he wanted her all over again.

Yet again, the tea went ignored.

The dogs woke them at eight, and she ran up to her flat and showered and dressed while Hugo let the dogs out.

He was in the shower when she came down, so she made coffee and put some toast in, then sat on the sofa, Lola's head on her lap and Rufus curled up under her arm, wondering what would happen next.

He hadn't outlined the rules beyond the 'don't do long-term' etc., but was she expected to move in with him? Sleep in her own bed unless and until either of them wanted to be together? 'The Rules', as she was starting to think of them, needed a little clarification. And maybe some of her own.

He appeared a few moments later, while her list was still a work in progress.

'Well, you all look comfy,' he said, and perched on the arm of the sofa, the only place left for him. 'I can smell coffee.'

'You can. And toast. It's only just done. Come on, dogs, shift, it's time for breakfast.'

The dogs leapt off the sofa, and Hugo stood and pulled her up into his arms. His hug was brief, and then he let her go and led the way into the kitchen, the dogs trotting at his heels.

After breakfast they walked the dogs along the beach, and as they headed back she broke the comfortable silence.

'What are your plans for the rest of the day?' she asked him, because it was that or wait for him to tell her.

'I don't really have any. I mean, there's always admin to do.'

'Well, while you're doing that, you can do a bill for Lola's treatment,' she told him, and raised an eyebrow when he opened his mouth.

He ignored the gesture. 'Don't you think we're rather past that?'

'Or I can do it myself.'

'So what are your plans?'

'First I need to go over to my house to make sure it's ready for my first booking. They're coming this afternoon.'

'Can I come?'

'Sure. You can give me your first impression of it.'

They let the dogs in, rubbed them down with towels to get the sand off their feet, and then headed over to her house on foot.

'It looks really good,' he told her as they walked round, and she smiled in relief.

'I did my best. I just hope they don't trash it.'

'Who is it, do you know?'

'A couple with a baby, and their parents, his or hers, I don't know.'

He chuckled. 'They don't sound like they'll trash it.'

'No, they don't. It was a good idea of yours.'

So long as nothing happened between them to upset the status quo. Not that she was entirely sure yet quite what that was…

* * *

They went back to the practice, and while Hugo busied himself in the office, she went food shopping.

She had to drop a welcome pack in for her tenants, so she picked up those things and some stuff for the barbecue. His idea, and of course because it was a glorious early May day, everyone else had the same idea and the shelves were a bit depleted.

She threw a selection of things into the basket, then detoured up the last aisle and dropped a packet of condoms in on the rest. Just in case…

By the time she'd been to the house and got back it was getting hotter, and she carried the food upstairs and then hesitated. His fridge or hers? Or both?

They definitely needed to lay down more rules…

Hugo heard her come in, and followed her upstairs.

'What did you get?'

'All sorts of stuff. I just don't know where to put it,' she told him, turning to meet his eyes. 'Are we living together? Cooking together? Sleeping together? Or living independently and meeting up for sex when the mood takes us? Are we lovers? Friends with benefits? What the hell are we, Hugo?'

He blinked at that. 'Wow. Um—are you OK, Ellie? Because that sounds…'

'Confused? Uncertain? I mean, you have all these *rules*, but they're so vague—'

'OK, so we have sex on Sunday evening, Tuesday lunchtime, Wednesday morning—oh, and we might cram a quickie in between consults—'

'Don't be sarcastic.'

He scrubbed a hand through his hair and sighed. 'I'm not being sarcastic, Ellie, and frankly, I don't know the answers either.' His voice gentled. 'And I don't know what we call this. I hate friends with benefits, it's—it's not what it is. It feels—I don't know, more than that. And I certainly don't want to call all the shots, that's not what this is about. Maybe we just need to be honest with each other, like say, *I want to spend the night alone*, or *Let's eat in mine tonight*, or…' he shrugged '… *I want you now.*'

She stared at him, her eyes searching. 'Do you?'

He felt his body react instantly, and he couldn't stop the little huff of laughter. He closed his eyes briefly. 'Of course I do. I always have done. Right from day one. But only if you do.'

She was still staring at him, something primal stirring in her eyes. Her lips parted, then shut, pursing a little. He could almost hear her mind work.

'Um—maybe we should put the food away

first?' she suggested after a sizzling pause, and he laughed and pulled her into his arms, folding her against his chest in a gentle hug.

'We probably should.'

Over the next few days, things sorted themselves out, because it turned out neither of them wanted to sleep alone, and it was easier with the dogs if they were in his flat rather than up the extra flight to hers.

And because they were there all the time, they cooked and ate in his kitchen, and hung out in his sitting room playing backgammon or watching TV or just talking about this and that.

Work was busier than usual, because people were going on holiday and so there were the usual panicked vaccinations that had been overlooked or forms to fill in for going abroad, and of course Kerry and James were on their honeymoon so they were a nurse down for that first week.

Then Kerry sent a group message, full of her honeymoon photos, both of them looking blissfully happy with life. And Ellie felt a pang of sadness that this wasn't ever going to be the case with her and Hugo.

Not in his rules. And yes, she understood where he was coming from, and in a way she was glad she knew where she stood with him, but underneath it all was an aching sadness that it couldn't be more, because she loved him.

She'd loved him since the day she'd met him, the day he saved Lola's life, and with every day she loved him more.

And he didn't do love.

So she kept smiling, got on with her work, and then on Thursday, just as she was about to take her lunch break, a client she'd seen before came in on the verge of tears. Ellie was in Reception at the time, and she ushered her into a consult room and closed the door.

'What's wrong?' she asked gently, because the dog looked absolutely fine, and her owner shook her head.

'My husband's—we've split up, and he doesn't want Bailey and I work full-time and I don't know where I'm going to live because I can't find a place I can afford where they allow dogs, and I can't leave him alone all day, and I can't work from home—'

'Do you want us to find a new home for him? Is that it?'

She nodded, fumbling in her pockets, and Ellie handed her a tissue. 'Thanks.'

She blew her nose and blinked away tears and met Ellie's eyes. 'It's just—he's such a lovely, gentle, kind dog, and I can't bear to think of him going to someone awful who doesn't understand dogs…'

'Let me talk to Hugo—in fact, hang on, if you can, and I'll see if he's free now?'

She went out the back into the corridor and heard his voice. He was in the office talking to Jean, and he looked up at her and broke off.

'Hi, what's up?'

'Client wants—no, she *needs* to rehome a dog. He's a Golden Retriever, three years old, absolutely lovely dog, they've split up and she can't find accommodation that'll allow her to keep him, she works full-time. I was thinking, Jenny?'

Jenny, who'd lost Nell in Ellie's first week, and was alone now.

'Who is he?'

'Mrs Williams' Bailey.'

'*Bailey?* I know Bailey, he'd be perfect for Jenny. Oh, she must be heartbroken. Is she still here with him?'

'Yes, she's in the consult room.'

'Jean, I'll be back. Ellie, let's go and talk to her.'

Bailey recognised him instantly and greeted him, tail wagging, smiling in the way that only a Golden Retriever could smile. He crouched down and gave him a fuss, then straightened up.

'I'm so sorry to hear about your circumstances, Mrs Williams. Are you OK to keep him a day or so while we make some enquiries? We have someone in mind, a lady who lost her dog recently who could be just right for him. She has grandchildren, and they visit her often and are used to dogs. They've had five over the years and she certainly knows what she's doing with them. I could call her? Would you mind?'

'Oh, could you? He loves children. I've got a baby nephew and he adores him, he's so gentle, and we thought…'

The tears started again, and it wasn't hard to work out why. A family dog, for a family that was never going to happen.

'I tell you what, why don't you stay here for a minute and let me go and make a call. OK?'

She nodded, and they left her there and went back to the office. Jean, reading his mind as ever, thrust a piece of paper at him.

'Jenny's number.'

'Thanks.' She picked up almost immediately, and after asking how she was, he said carefully, 'Look, I know it's still early days, but have you given any thought to getting another dog?'

'Oh, Hugo—I don't know. The house just feels so *wrong* without a dog, but I can't cope with a puppy right now, and an older rescue dog might come with all sorts of issues.'

'How about a three-year-old Golden Retriever? Lovely boy, sweet, friendly, gentle dog, loves everybody, good with children, fit and healthy, and needs a new home through no fault of his own. Change of personal circumstances, but he's very much loved.'

'Oh, poor boy, he sounds… Oh, Hugo, I don't know. Is he with you?'

'He is at the moment.'

There was a long pause, then she said, 'Can I come now?'

'Sure. Come to the back door, you can meet him in the office.'

They sent Mrs Williams back to the waiting room and took Bailey through to the office, put Lola and Rufus in the kennels out of the way, and after a very few minutes Jenny arrived.

Hugo met her at the back door and ushered her in, and she took one look at Bailey and fell in love.

'Oh, the dear, dear boy…'

'Here, have a seat.' He turned a chair round and she sat on it and held out a hand, and the dog came over and licked it and sat beside her and leant against her leg, his head tilted up, staring at her as if she was his best friend.

'Oh, he's such a sweetheart… He reminds me of Rupert.'

'I'm sure he can be naughty.'

Jenny laughed and looked up at him, smiling the first real smile he'd seen on her in months. 'Hugo, all dogs can be naughty. It's part of their charm. Nell was still naughty. Oh, the poor, sweet boy. Can I ask why?'

'Divorce, and she works full-time.'

'Oh, no, that wouldn't work, Goldens need all

the love all the time. Oh, Bailey. Are you a good boy? Are you?'

Bailey wagged his tail, tongue lolling, a silly smile on his face, and that was it. 'I'll take him.'

'Are you sure? You don't have to make a decision now. Do you want to think about it?'

She looked up and met his eyes. 'Hugo, I've thought about nothing else since Nell, and she would have loved him. I don't need to think any more. I want to take him home as soon as I can.'

'Let me fetch his owner. I'm sure she'd love to meet you.'

Half an hour later a tearful Mrs Williams said goodbye to Bailey and left him with his new owner. He whined for a moment, but a bit of a cuddle and a gravy bone treat brought him back to Jenny.

'She's left a bag of his toys and blankets in Reception, and also his bed, so you can take them home with you. I'll give you a hand out to the car.'

He saw her off, then went back inside and found Ellie up to her eyes with consults, and he took some of them off her.

Jo, their Thursday vet, was busy doing the first of two dentals, and Ellie was in dire need of a break. So was he, but hey, he was the boss.

'Are you sure you've got time? I thought you were busy with Jenny.'

'No, she's gone home with Bailey. Go and eat

something, and after we've finished tonight we'll take the dogs for a walk by the river and go to the pub.'

It was a lovely walk, the dogs enjoying the change of scenery as much as she was, and she breathed in deeply and sighed. 'There's something so evocative about the smell of river mud at low tide,' she murmured, and Hugo chuckled.

'Only when it's in the river. When it's on the dogs it's less great.'

She laughed, picturing the two of them if they'd been off the lead. They couldn't be, of course, because of the ground-nesting wetland birds, but they were still having fun.

'So how did it go with Jenny?'

'Oh, she's in love. I think they'll be fine. She knows what she's doing.'

Ellie didn't reply. She was busy thinking about the comparison between them, Jenny in love with Bailey, who wouldn't have any rules or restrictions on the breadth and depth of her love for him, and her, falling deeper and deeper in love with an enigmatic loner with a broken heart and a rule book that lay between them like a minefield.

What on earth was she doing with him? Unlike Jenny with Bailey, she didn't have a clue. She just knew it was bound to end in tears…

CHAPTER NINE

FRIDAY WAS AS hectic as ever, and as soon as all her consults were done, she headed over to her house.

Her tenants had left this morning, and a new family were coming in tomorrow. She opened the front door with a feeling of trepidation, but the house was immaculate, and there was a note on the worktop thanking her for a lovely break and saying they'd like to book again later in the summer.

They'd be more than welcome. The bathroom and kitchen had both been cleaned, the beds stripped and the carpeted floors vacuumed, so there wasn't much for her to do. She put on the fresh bedding, ran a duster round the house, emptied the dishwasher and then headed back to Hugo.

She found him in his kitchen, busy stirring something on the hob, and she wrapped her arms round him and peered down into the pan. Chilli? 'That smells delicious.'

'Hopefully. So how was the house?'

'Brilliant. I couldn't believe it. They'd cleaned everything.'

'Wow. That's good. So when do your next tenants come?'

'Tomorrow afternoon, and they're here till Wednesday. I'll need to pop over first thing tomorrow with a welcome pack before we start. Then I've got another family from next Saturday for two weeks. Have the dogs been out?'

'Yes. Not far, but they've been out in the garden quite a bit today. They get on really well. Oh, and I heard from Jenny. Bailey cried a bit in the night, but then he settled and she's really happy. She brought us some chocolates as a thank you.'

She rolled her eyes. 'More chocolates? We'll all be obese and diabetic.'

He threw her a wry grin. 'Don't worry about that, some days it's all that keeps us going. I have to say I'm glad Kerry's back on Monday, we've been picking up all sorts of things she usually does, so we might get time to eat actual food.'

It was a vain hope.

They were every bit as busy, and the week flew by. She went over late on Wednesday to get her house ready for the new people coming on Saturday, and then on Friday afternoon, as it was all winding down at the end of the day, Lucy walked in via the back door with her baby in her arms, and everyone who could downed tools and congregated in the office for a look at the new arrival.

Ellie was still busy while they were all cooing over baby Freya, but when she emerged after her last consult ended, she went in there for a peek.

'Oh, she's gorgeous,' she said softly, just as Hugo walked in, and Lucy laughed.

'She'd be more gorgeous if she slept through the night. Hey, Hugo, do me a favour and hold her while I nip to the loo?'

And without waiting for an answer, she dumped Freya into his arms.

For a fleeting second he looked paralysed, then Freya cried and instinct kicked in and he shifted her gently into a better position, smiling at her and murmuring reassuring nothings to soothe her, and Ellie stared at him, gazing down at Freya with such tenderness that she wanted to cry.

And then he looked up and met her eyes.

For a moment he froze, his face filled with longing, a deep yearning he'd never let her see before, and then his eyes went blank as the shutters came down. He turned away and walked out, still talking to Freya, but away from Ellie, away from the others.

Lucy appeared, and he handed Freya back instantly.

'Has she been OK?'

'Fine. Sorry, got to go. Congratulations, she's beautiful.'

He dropped a kiss on her cheek and walked away, heading for the door to his flat with Rufus at his heels, leaving Ellie standing there staring at the space where he'd been. She'd thought he was OK until he'd looked up, and then she'd seen the longing in his eyes—for Samuel, or for a child he'd never let himself have?

Oh, Hugo. Had that shown in her own eyes? The ache in her heart for him, and for a child of his that she'd never be able to hold?

Or the ache in his own heart, reflected back at him…

She needed to go to him.

He turned the latch on his door, went upstairs and locked the door to the back stairs, then walked into the sitting room and dropped onto the sofa.

He could still smell the baby—that evocative, unforgettable mixture of milk and nappy cream.

How? How can I remember that?

How could he forget?

He closed his eyes to shut out the images, but it didn't work. Of course it didn't work.

And nor did this thing he had going with Ellie. He'd been OK until she'd rocked up in his life and invaded the safe little cocoon he'd built around himself. He'd let her in because he couldn't help himself, but he couldn't do it any more, couldn't let her stay there, knocking down the protective walls around his heart brick by brick with every kiss, every touch, because he knew what would come next.

He'd seen the need in her eyes, the longing he could never dare to fulfil. It was a longing that was all too familiar to him, but Samuel was gone and he'd never get him back—

He heard her on the back stairs, the rattle of the door handle, the knock.

'Hugo? Hugo, let me in.'

Rufus ran to the door and scratched at it, whining, and he closed his eyes.

'Hugo, please, don't do this. We need to talk.'

She was right, they did.

And he knew exactly what he had to say…

Ellie rested her head against the door, her heart pounding, dread running through her veins.

Why wouldn't he talk to her? Why—

She heard the key turn, and the door opened.

Oh, Hugo...

He looked awful, jaw clenched, eyes blank and yet not. He turned away and she followed him into the sitting room. He walked straight past the sofa where they sat each night, over to the window, staring through it as if he was looking for something.

Words?

'Hugo, please talk to me.'

He turned, hands still rammed in his pockets,

his back to the light, and she sat down on the arm of the sofa as if her strings were cut.

He was going to end it. She couldn't read the expression on his face but she didn't need to, she could see it in every defensive line of his body.

'We can't do this any more. You're getting in too deep, and I can't let you do that. I don't want it, and if you had any sense, nor would you. You deserve better. You deserve someone who can give you what you need, give you a family, a stable home life, the love you deserve, and that's never going to be me.'

No...

'Why don't you let me be the judge of what I need?'

'Because your judgement's clouded. Yes, the sex is great, but that's all it is, all it could ever be.'

'You're wrong, Hugo. I don't care about the sex, it's neither here nor there. It's way more than that—'

'Only for you. And I don't want it any more.' He closed his eyes and she saw him swallow. 'I can't love you, Ellie. And you need a man who will. A man who *can*.'

She stood up, legs shaking like jelly, and took a step towards him, but he held up his hand to ward her off.

'Don't—'

Don't what? Don't go and put your arms around him and tell him you love him? Don't tell him he's all you'll ever need, that you don't care about having a family, so long as you have him?

His face blurred, but for a few more seconds she stood her ground, and then she sucked in a breath and drew herself up. She wasn't going to grovel.

'Goodbye, Hugo,' she said softly.

And then she turned and walked out of his flat, her heart in shreds. Lola was torn between the two of them, and she called her, closing the door behind them and heading up the stairs on trembling legs.

Seven weeks. Seven weeks today since she'd hit the road and driven here, into his life. How was it only that?

She reached her flat and closed the door, somehow holding it together, her heart numb. She knew it wouldn't stay that way, but for now, she had to escape from here and get as far away from him as she could before the tears came.

She packed her things—not all of them, she didn't have enough bags or enough energy. Just the things she and Lola would need.

She carried it all downstairs, put it into her car, came back for Lola's bed, her food, her toys, and then put Lola in the car and drove away.

Hugo stood at the window and watched her go, his eyes dry, his heart thudding against his ribcage.

He'd done the right thing, for her, for him.

The only thing.

He just hadn't expected it to hurt quite so much.

His chest heaved and he fought down the sob, but it tore its way out of his chest anyway. He walked into his bedroom and lay on the bed, but it smelt of her, the lingering trace of her scent wrapping around him, engulfing him in pain.

Rufus whined and licked his face, and he realised tears were leaking out of the corners of his eyes and dribbling down onto the pillow. He let them fall. He owed her that, at least…

She didn't know where to go.

Her house? Too close, and anyway she had holidaymakers arriving tomorrow.

Oh, no. Welcome pack.

She pulled over into the forecourt of a mini-supermarket, left Lola in the car and grabbed a few things—milk, teabags, bread, butter, eggs, cheese, biscuits, jam—just something to tide them over after a journey—and dropped them off at the house.

Seven weeks ago today, almost to the hour, she'd let Lola out into the garden and she'd been injured. Seven short weeks that had been the best and worst weeks of her life.

And now here she was again, back to square one, only now with an intact dog and a broken heart.

Where could she go?

Nowhere, at this time of night, but she couldn't stay here in Yoxburgh. Too close, too many memories of Hugo.

So she locked the house, left the key in the key safe she'd had installed and drove away.

Instinct and adrenaline got her down the A12 and round the M25, and then a near-miss as she went up the slip road and onto the M40 brought her to her senses. She drove to the motel she'd stayed at before, checked into a dog-friendly room and fed Lola, then lay on the bed, dry-eyed, cast adrift once more on the sea of life without a rudder or a compass to guide her, the future a yawning void…

Where could she go? What should she do?

Somehow she slept, Lola on the bed beside her, and when she woke it was just gone five. Too early for breakfast, not that she was hungry, but she fed Lola, picked up her bag, clipped her on her lead and left the room, dropping her key in the slot on her way out.

She drove on autopilot, and shortly after six she turned onto Jim's drive and cut the engine. The light was on in his kitchen. Of course it was, because her old boss and mentor had always been an early riser and the kettle would be on. His face appeared in the window, then the front door opened and he stood there, a familiar silhouette in a world that seemed suddenly alien.

She got out of the car and walked towards him,

and he took one look at her and held out his arms. She fell into them, felt the warmth and strength of them close around her, holding her safe, and felt herself starting to fall apart.

'Oh, dear, dear girl. Come inside and have a cup of tea.'

'Lola,' she said, and he let the dog out of the car and brought her inside, ushering Ellie into the kitchen.

'This one looks as if she could do with a run in the garden, and you look as if you could do with a nice cup of tea,' he said, and while he opened the back door and took Lola outside, she sat down at his kitchen table where she'd sat so many times before, and finally, finally, the tears fell.

He didn't say a word when he came back in with Lola, just put a mug down on the table in front of her and handed her a wad of tissues.

'I'm sorry,' she managed, sniffing and scrubbing at her eyes, but he squeezed her hand briefly.

'No need to apologise. You're safe here, and you don't have to tell me anything.'

Just as well, because right then she was beyond making any sense. She cradled the mug, warming her ice-cold hands on it, but she didn't drink.

'I should have rung—'

'Nonsense. My door's always open to you, Ellie. You know that. I wish you'd come to me before.'

So did she, now, looking back, but then she'd

never have met Hugo, never known just how beautiful love could be.

Or how painful.

The tears welled again, and she swiped at them, her hands shaking.

'When did you last eat anything?'

She stared blankly at him. 'Eat…? I—I don't remember, Jim. Maybe lunch yesterday? I'm not sure, maybe a chocolate? I had a biscuit in the motel last night, but—no, not really.'

She wasn't even making sense, but Jim just tutted softly and got up and put some bread in the toaster, took eggs out of a bowl and a pan from the rack and cracked the eggs into it, added milk, a knob of butter, a twist of salt and pepper, beat them together and set them on the hob while he buttered the toast.

Moments later he put their two plates down on the table and sat down.

'Come on, eat up,' he told her, pushing the plate of scrambled eggs towards her, and she suddenly realised how hungry she was.

She ate, and then when she'd finished every last morsel, Jim cleared the plates away, sat down again and met her eyes.

'Is this about Hugo?'

The kindness and sympathy in his eyes were too much for her, so she looked down at her hands, finding a crumb on the table and pushing it around with her fingertip until she couldn't see it any longer.

'I should have known better,' she said unevenly. 'God knows he warned me, Jim. He told me it wasn't going anywhere, and he gave me a whole list of rules, things he didn't do, like permanent or long-term or love, said he didn't make promises he couldn't keep—and I somehow managed to forget all about that and fall in love with him anyway—'

Jim's firm, kindly hand closed over hers and gave it a gentle squeeze.

'I'm so sorry. I thought you'd be all right with Hugo, I thought he'd take care of you.'

'Oh, he did. He was so kind, so decent, so—and he still is, Jim. That's the awful thing. It's not about us, it's about—'

She sucked in a shaky breath. 'He had a baby. Ten years ago, and he was born with a chromosomal disorder that was incompatible with life, and he died when he was eight weeks old. And it broke him, Jim. It broke him more than I'd realised. I suppose I thought at first I could stick to his stupid rules, but then I couldn't, I went and fell in love with him, and still I thought we'd be OK, and then… I'm—no, I *was* covering someone's maternity leave, and she brought her baby in, and she's about the same age as his baby was, I guess, and she gave her to him to hold, and the way he looked at her, the tenderness, the longing—I just wanted to cry for him, and then he saw my face, and…'

'And?'

'I went after him, asked him to talk to me, and he told me it was over, he didn't love me, he told me I needed to go and find a nice man and have babies with him, but I don't want to have babies with a nice man, I want to have babies with Hugo, and if I can't have babies, well, tough, but I want him, I love him, and he won't even give us a chance—'

The tears erupted again, and she felt Jim's hand on her shoulder giving it a gentle squeeze.

'Oh, dear, oh, dear. I'm so sorry, Ellie. Love can be a hard thing to bear at times.'

And then she felt a wave of guilt because Marion, his wife of more than forty years, was in a care home and didn't know who he was any more.

She scrubbed away the tears and looked at him. 'How's Marion?'

'Oh, you know. Some days are better than others. But it is what it is, and we put one foot in front of the other and keep on going. That's what it's all about, isn't it?'

Was that what Hugo had been doing for the last ten years, putting one foot in front of the other? And then she'd come along and upset the fragile equilibrium of his life, and it had all come tumbling down on top of them.

'I'm so sorry. I shouldn't be here, you've got enough to deal with.'

He laid a hand on Lola's head, and Ellie realised she'd left her side and was leaning against his leg as if to comfort him. She looked around, puzzled, but there was no sign…

'Jim, where's Milo?' she asked softly, knowing the answer but not ready to believe it.

'He died—a month ago. His heart. I found him in the morning, curled up in his bed asleep. And the house doesn't feel the same without him or Marion.'

Like Jenny, when she'd lost her beloved Nell so soon after George. And now there was Bailey…

'Do you think you'll get another dog?'

He gave a soft, humourless little laugh. 'I'm not sure I've got the stamina for it, or the time. I spend most days with Marion—not that she realises, half the time. But I do, and I'm there because she's still my wife and I still love her.'

Of course he did—and she still loved Hugo. The difference was Hugo knew exactly who she was and he didn't want her there, didn't want her love…

'He may come round, you know.'

She could have laughed at that. 'Hugo? No. He's too—oh, gosh. Principled? Decent? He really seems to believe that being a mother is what I'm on the earth for, and it's not, or not the only thing. I'm thirty-two, Jim, and this is the first time I've ever met anyone I loved enough to even consider having a child with. And now it's not even for me, it's for Hugo.'

'Having another baby won't bring his dead baby back, Ellie. Was it planned, do you know?'

She shook her head. 'No. They were off and on, as he put it, and it was just a tragic accident. And it's broken him, Jim. He said he'll never have another child, and he'd be such a good father.'

'Maybe he doesn't want to be? Not everyone's cut out for it.'

'You've got four and I don't remember you complaining,' she reminded him, and he gave a rueful chuckle.

'No, and we've three grandchildren, now, and I wouldn't change it for the world, but if it hadn't happened for us, we would still have been happy together.'

'Maybe I should give you his number so you can tell him that.'

'It's not me that has to tell him that, Ellie. It's you. But not yet. Let the dust settle. Stay here, you and Lola, for as long as you need, and then when you're ready, go and talk to him.'

'He won't talk. He's got a stubborn streak a mile wide.'

'He's not alone in that. Don't give up on him yet, Ellie. Give him time. He'll be missing you, too.'

How could he miss her so much?

He hadn't slept all night—changing the sheets had got rid of her scent, but it didn't do anything for the memories of her lying there with him. So he'd got up and gone down to the office and changed the rota, emailed Jo and asked her to do Saturday morning, juggled things around later in the week so he or Jo were picking up the times Ellie would have been in surgery, then he took Rufus out for a run at stupid o'clock, ran for an hour and came back and showered, sent Jo a text to be sure she'd got his message, and then went downstairs to get on with the day.

Thank goodness it was only Saturday and he didn't have a full day of electives to fit in, but that didn't really help his mood. He was terse with everyone, and Kerry took him on one side after a short while and told him to get a grip or they'd all be leaving.

'It's not their fault you and Ellie have had a row—'

'We haven't had a row. She had to go away.'

'Had to? Is that why you're like a bear with a sore head? I wasn't born yesterday. You've obviously split up—'

'We weren't together—'

'Oh, come on, Hugo, tell it to the fairies! It's been blindingly obvious since the wedding. Everybody knows.'

'Nothing happened at the wedding.'

'Oh, don't give me that. The way you two were dancing? There was only one place you were going when you left—and don't bother to deny it. So why's she gone? What did you say to her?'

'It's none of your business, Kerry.'

'It's my business when you upset my nurses.'

He scraped a hand through his hair and gave a sharp sigh. 'I told her to go. She's left.'

'*Left?* You mean she's not coming back?'

'No. She's not coming back.'

Kerry stared at him for an age, then light dawned in her eyes and her voice softened. 'Oh, Hugo… This is because of Lucy's baby, isn't it?'

He swallowed hard. 'Don't go there, Kerry, please.'

'Oh, Hugo…'

She hugged him hard, then told him to go. 'You don't need to be here. We can manage, Jo's in, she can do the consults. I'll shut up shop. Go and see Peter and Sally. Talk to them.'

'I can't just leave you all—'

'You can. Seriously, we can cope and you're no use to us anyway like this. Go.'

So he went, taking Rufus with him and leaving the practice in Kerry's very capable hands. Not that he had the slightest clue what to say to his godparents when he turned up on the doorstep at ten on a Saturday morning, but it turned out he didn't have to.

'Come in, Hugo,' Peter said, and he walked in and found Sally in the kitchen.

'Oh, you're here, darling. Sit down, coffee'll be ready in a minute. Would you like something to eat?'

'No, I'm—I'm fine.'

'Are you? Because you don't look it.' She pointed to a chair. 'Sit down, you're cluttering the place up. I'll make some toast.'

The light dawned. 'Kerry rang you, didn't she?'

'She might have done.'

'Interfering—'

'She's got your best interests at heart, Hugo,' Peter said quietly. 'We all have. And we're here if you need to talk.'

'I don't want to talk,' he said tightly. 'There's nothing to say. She's gone. End of.'

'Because of the baby?' Sally, this time, not knowing when to leave well alone. What was it with the women in his life?

'You, too? It's nothing to do with Lucy's baby—'

'I wasn't talking about Lucy's baby, Hugo,' she said softly. 'I was talking about Samuel.'

He felt himself flinch and looked away.

'So what happened with Ellie?'

She wasn't going to give up, but then nor was he.

She plonked a plate of hot buttered toast in the middle of the table, poured the coffee and sat down, waiting.

He picked up a slice of toast and bit into it, but he could hardly swallow past the tightness of his throat. He gave up and put it down again.

'Lucy came in with Freya, and I thought I ought to show my face, and she just handed her to me and went to the loo. And then Freya cried, and I—just knew what to do. It all came back, and the smell—it was so familiar, so—'

'So what happened then?'

'Ellie was looking at me, and her face—' He broke off and looked down, poking at the slice of toast for something to do, crumbling it into little bits between his fingers. 'She doesn't need me. She needs someone to give her children. She'd be a brilliant mother. She *needs* to be a mother.'

'And you need to be a father.'

'No. I've *been* a father. I *am* a father. Never again.'

'Why? Why, when you were so good with Samuel?'

'*Because* of him. I don't want—don't want to overlay my memories. I don't want to forget—'

His voice cracked, and he felt Sally's hand on his shoulder.

'You'll never forget him,' she said gently. 'He'll live in you for ever, Hugo. That's what happens, but it doesn't mean you can't try again—and even if you don't, even if you never have children, you'd have each other.'

She took Peter's hand and squeezed it, and he covered her hand with his.

'We were never blessed with children,' he said quietly, 'it just never happened for us, but there's no way we'd rather not have been together. We've had a wonderful life, we've been together for forty-five years, and we're still in love. And if we'd known at the start that one of us couldn't have a child, there's no way it would have made the slightest difference to how much we love each other and want to be together.'

'You weren't really childless, though, were you? You were lumbered with me—'

'We were never *lumbered* with you,' Sally said firmly. 'We were more than happy to have you, and you've brought so much richness into our lives, but even without you, we would still have felt the same. It isn't children that make a marriage, Hugo, it's love, first and foremost.'

'But—what if she really wanted a baby? What if she got pregnant? I can't—I'm not brave enough.'

'They said it was a one-off,' Peter reminded him.

'But it could be something else next time. I can't lose anyone else—'

'You've lost Ellie. Doesn't that matter?'

He sucked in a breath. 'Of course it matters! But a child—it would just open the wound…'

'Which will never heal unless you let it, Hugo,' Sally said softly, taking his hands in hers. 'You need to let yourself grieve.'

He snatched his hands back.

'Don't tell me about grief, Sally. I know enough about grief. I could write a book about it.'

'You've never grieved for Samuel. You just threw yourself back into work and carried on, business as usual—except it wasn't, was it? That's why you've worked so hard, spent all your time keeping busy, and you've never really let yourself love anyone since your parents died.'

'That's not true, I love you.'

'You already loved us, just as we loved you.'

They had. 'I was horrible to you.'

'You'd just lost your parents! That's huge. And we understood, of course we did, but you've never had a serious relationship, and ever since Samuel you've sabotaged anything that might lead to love. And now it's even worse, because you've found someone to love and you've sent her away. You're just hiding from your grief, Hugo, and you've been doing it ever since he died.'

Had he?

He pushed back his chair. 'I don't need to listen to this—'

'Maybe not, but maybe it's time to listen to your heart.'

CHAPTER TEN

He drove away, no fixed idea of where he was going, just anywhere away from the people who loved him and thought it was their business to sort him out.

If only it were that easy.

He couldn't go back to the practice while they were all there, so he drove down to the harbour, parked the car and took Rufus for a walk. Not that he needed one, not after their run that he'd thought was a good idea well before dawn. He had no idea what time he'd left or how long they'd run for, but he'd been back at five thirty and he'd felt wiped.

Still did, but he couldn't rest, couldn't settle to anything, so he walked, until Rufus finally sat down and refused to move. He sat beside him on the edge of the path, legs resting on the bank down to the river, the smell of the estuary reminding him of Ellie.

He'd walked here with her and Lola, the day

Jenny had taken Bailey home because she missed Nell and she missed George.

He sighed, and laid a hand on Rufus.

'I miss her, Rufe,' he said softly. 'I had to let her go, but I miss her.' Just another ache, another loss to carry with him.

He blinked to clear his vision and got to his feet, picking up the exhausted Rufus and carrying him back to the car.

Listen to your heart.

That was what Sally had said to him, but he had no idea what it was trying to say. All he could hear was all the reasons why he'd done the right thing letting her go.

Had he?

Although actually he hadn't *let* her go, he'd sent her away. And he'd lied to her, but he'd do it again if she came back.

He'd have to, for her sake, because she wanted something he could never give her.

He drove away from the harbour on autopilot, turned off and found himself somewhere he hadn't been for ten years, his heart apparently leading him where he needed to go. He drove slowly into the almost empty car park and stopped the engine.

'Come on, Rufus, let's go for a little walk. It's not far.'

He clipped his lead on, and they left the car park and wandered along the pretty, tree-lined path. It led between gravestones, some ancient, others newer, and then it came to another area, set aside from the rest, with tiny headstones set among the bobbing heads of wildflowers coming into bloom.

His feet led him in the right direction, and he knelt down in front of the simple headstone and laid his hand gently on the grass.

Maybe it's time to listen to your heart.

He didn't have a choice. It was beating so hard it was deafening, but it brought him no answers.

Why?

But nothing answered his silent scream. Rufus leant against him, and he sat down cross-legged and pulled him onto his lap and held him against his flailing heart while he let the memories flood in.

Samuel, his poor body compromised, his brave little heart doing its best against impossible odds, but his eyes would look up as clear as day, follow you, watch you. He'd recognised people, would turn towards the voices of the people he knew, kick his legs in delight, and sometimes he'd reward them with a smile. He loved to be sung to, would listen intently to voices, react to their tone.

He remembered singing to him, an old-fashioned lullaby his mother had sung him as a child. He used to sing it to him every night, and Samuel had loved it. He'd sung it to him softly as he lay dying in his arms…

He hummed it now, rocking gently, his hand still lying on the grass, and as he sang his heart slowed and steadied. Yes, it still ached, and it always would, but coming here, singing that tender lullaby, had reminded him of the good things that he'd forgotten.

He stayed there an age, lost in his memories, until Rufus started to fidget. He had no idea how long he'd been there, but Rufus was telling him it was time to go, and he unfolded his legs and got stiffly to his knees, kissing his fingers and pressing them to the grass where his baby lay, surrounded by all the other little ones who'd gone too young.

'I'm sorry I've been such a rubbish father. I should have come before, but I'll come again soon, I promise. I love you.'

He slept that night, then spent the next day going through his photos, printing some out and framing them. He propped them on the bookcase in his study with the one of himself with his parents, and put one, his favourite, on his bedside table.

The memories still tore him apart, but in a good way, now, and he realised just how much of himself he'd shut away for the last ten years since Samuel died.

And on Monday morning, he apologised to all the staff.

'I've not been in a good place—that's nothing new, I've not been in a good place for a long time, but Saturday was—well, anyway, I'm sorry. Sorry I took it out on you when it was nothing to do with any of you, but it won't happen again.'

There were a few murmurs, and then one of the junior nurses said cautiously, 'Is Ellie coming back?'

He swallowed hard. 'I don't know. Probably not. But I'm going to start advertising in earnest for a new vet, and I'm going to try and get a locum in the meantime, and until then I guess we all need to work a bit harder, but I'll do my best to sort it.'

More murmuring, and then, realising he'd finished, they went back to their tasks.

'Well done.' Kerry patted his shoulder on the way past, and Jean met his eyes.

'Are you really all right?'

He smiled. 'As all right as I can be.'

'Peter rang. He said he could come and help out if we need him.'

Hugo swallowed hard. 'I think we'll be OK, Jean. I'll give him a call.'

He sent him a quick message, and then there in his messaging app was Ellie's photo. He was so tempted to message her, but he needed to get his head straight before he could do that.

She couldn't ignore it any longer.

She'd been with Jim for two weeks, and there'd

been nothing from Hugo. Not that she'd expected to hear from him, but she'd hoped…

Would he talk to her now? Hear what she had to say? Because if these weeks away from him had proved one thing, it was that she couldn't live without him. And if that meant they never had a family, well, so be it. Lots of people were in that situation, some because it had never happened for them, others by choice.

And it could be their choice.

Jim was with Marion, so she wasn't able to talk to him, but she wrote him a note thanking him for all his kindness and understanding and promising to be in touch, and then she stripped her bed, packed up all their things and loaded them and Lola into the car.

Her tenants would have left this morning and she'd kept the next two weeks clear, so if all else failed she could live at her house while she worked out what to do with her life, but for now, at least, she wasn't giving up on Hugo.

He needed her every bit as much as she needed him, and she knew—she just *knew*—that he loved her. He'd lied to protect her, and for that she loved him even more, but she had to convince him that it wasn't necessary. She didn't need protecting, she needed him. Nothing else.

She was on the M25 when her phone tinged, but it was probably nothing, so she ignored it until she got to the South Mimms service area at the

A1 junction. She found a space, dug her phone out of her bag and glanced at it.

Hugo?

She tapped to open it, her heart pounding.

Where are you?

She stared at it, the text blurring, her heart trying to escape from her chest. Why did he want to know?

She struggled to get her shaking fingers to work.

On M25. Why?

His reply was instant.

Need to talk to you.

To say what? She had no idea. She hesitated, then:

I'm on my way back.

Come on, Hugo…

Drive carefully. Call me when you get here.

She got Lola out of the car, her legs shaking, her whole body trembling, and led her to a patch of grass at the edge of the car park.

He wants to talk...

Her heart was pounding so hard she could hardly think, and she couldn't drive like this. She needed a drink and something to eat, so she put Lola back in the car, ran into the services, bought a bottle of water and a sandwich and ran back out. She shared the water with Lola, and sat in the car and took a bite of the sandwich and made herself swallow it, and the next one, and the next, until her heart had slowed a little.

Then she screwed the lid back on the water, put her seat belt on and headed back onto the M25.

Hugo sat on the sofa, staring at his phone.

She's coming back. Why?

Tenant change-over day, he realised. Of course.

His heart sank. For a moment there he'd thought…

No. He'd told her he didn't want her, didn't love her. Who in their right mind would want to talk to him again?

But maybe…

He went shopping. Just in case. He knew exactly what he was going to buy, and he had the recipe on his phone to remind him.

He found everything he needed, went home, did all the necessary prep and followed the recipe meticulously. And then, when it was done, he turned the heat off under the casserole dish, closed the kitchen door and went into the study, stood at the window and waited for her car to appear.

She turned into the practice, parked the car and sat there, her heart in her mouth.

Lola was standing up, tail thrashing, and she got out of the car and unclipped her harness. She shot out of the car, lead trailing, and ran straight up to Rufus, who was wagging furiously in delight.

And then she looked past them, and there was Hugo.

He looked drawn, thinner, his mouth unsmiling, and she walked towards him, her legs like jelly.

'You made good time,' he said.

It was the last thing she'd expected him to say, and her heart sank. Until she saw the muscle clenching in his jaw, and realised his heart was beating so hard she could see the pulse at his throat.

She walked up to him and then stopped, not knowing how to greet him or what to say. He saved her the trouble.

'Let's go up to my flat. I've cooked for us,' he said, and led the way.

She followed him, all her carefully rehearsed speeches forgotten. This was Hugo's gig, she'd let him do the talking.

For now.

* * *

He didn't know what to say, where to start. Except…

'I'm sorry.'

They were on the sofa in his sitting room, the room where two weeks ago he'd told her to leave. Told her he didn't love her. Told her to go and find a nice man and make babies with him.

Her eyes were fixed on his, searching.

'What for?'

'Lying to you. I said I didn't want you in my life any more, but it was a lie. I told myself I was trying to protect you, but I wasn't, I was trying to protect myself, and I wasn't ready to acknowledge the truth.'

'And now?'

'And now, I am. I've spent the last two weeks sorting my head out, dealing with a lot of stuff I should have dealt with years ago.' He took a breath. 'Losing Samuel was brutal. It broke my heart, and so I shut down and I didn't let myself feel any more. I didn't want to feel, didn't want to love. I just wanted to carry on being numb, because it was safe.

'What happened after the wedding really shouldn't have happened. I wasn't ready for what it made me feel, and I couldn't handle it. I hadn't dealt with Samuel's death—hell, I probably hadn't dealt with my parents' deaths, and I've never let myself love anyone. I've avoided it like the plague because I couldn't bear to expose myself to losing anyone else. And then you came along and blew all that out the water, and it scared the hell out of me.

'You'd broken through my defences, and you made me want more in my life than I could bear, more than was safe. And so I lashed out, because I was afraid of unleashing all the feelings I'd denied for the last ten years.

'I didn't mean to love you, but I did, and I hadn't even realised. It hit me like a train, and I was scared. I was so scared. And I'm so sorry I hurt you.'

'So what now?' she asked, her face guarded, but she wasn't giving anything away and he had no idea where she was in her head. He could only hope.

'That's all down to you,' he said, and waited.

And then finally, she spoke.

'I thought I could cope with us being friends,' she said quietly, 'but I wanted more. I'd never found anyone I could trust with my heart, and then I met you, and you were so kind, so caring, so generous, and I thought I might be safe with you, that you wouldn't leave me like my father left my mother…' Her voice cracked and she swallowed, then went on, 'I thought you were different. And then you sent me away.'

His face creased with pain. 'Oh, Ellie… I only

did it for you. I was too scared of the future, too scared we might lose a child, and I knew you wanted children. The way you looked at me when I was holding Freya—the longing. And I felt it, too, and I just couldn't deal with it.'

'So what's different now?' she asked, her heart pounding as she waited for his answer. She could see the sincerity in his eyes, but could she trust it?

'I am. I told Sally and Peter I was afraid of losing anyone else, and Sally pointed out I'd lost you anyway. And she was right. I had, and it left this yawning void…'

'So—what now, Hugo?'

'I want you back.'

'Really?' she asked, pushing him for the truth. 'For ever, or just for this week? Because right now you're sounding a lot like my father apparently did and I'm not sure I can dare to believe anything you tell me.'

His eyes prickled and he turned away. 'I guess I deserve that.'

'So why do you really need me back? Because you need a locum?'

He stared at her, shocked that she could even think that, but then what had he ever done that might make her think differently?

'Absolutely not. I have a locum. What I don't have is you, Ellie, and I love you, and I'm lost without you.'

* * *

His voice cracked, and she stared at him, searching his eyes, so readable now, if she only dared to trust what they were telling her.

'You really want me back?'

'Yes.'

'What, just to take up where we left off?'

'No—well, yes, but—no.'

'Hugo, you're not making any sense. Do you want me back, or do you not want me back?'

'Yes, I do want you back. Of course I want you back!'

'OK. And what about your rules?'

He looked puzzled. 'My rules?'

'"I don't do long term, I don't do—"'

He held up his hand. 'No rules—well, that's not quite true. There is one. We tell the truth. Always. And the truth is, I love you, and I want to be with you.'

Could it really be so easy?

No. It never was, and they'd only had nine weeks to get to this point, and they'd been apart for two of them.

'You honestly love me?'

'Yes, Ellie. I honestly love you. Honestly and truly and with all my heart, tattered though it is. And no, I'm not perfect, I know that, but I promise I'll do my best not to hurt you ever again.'

Her eyes were welling up, but she blinked hard and pulled herself together.

'And no rules? Because I don't want to get in any deeper and have you change your mind because you realise that actually you *don't* do long term after all.'

He smiled, a rueful flicker of his lips, a softening of his eyes. 'No rules. Only the truth.'

She swallowed, looked away, looked back at him.

'And this stuff you had to deal with…?'

His smile faded. 'Ah. When I went to see Peter and Sally, Sally pointed out I'd never let myself grieve for Samuel, never let myself move on. I'd cut myself off from any joy, any love—until I met you. And then I still wouldn't let it in. And then I lost you and everything seemed pointless—my work, my life—all of it. I went to Samuel's grave, and I talked to him, and then I came home and I cried. I'd never cried for him—'

'Oh, Hugo…'

She reached out to him, and then she was in his arms, and he was holding her close, his lips pressed against her cheek, and she tilted her head back and met his eyes. 'Are you OK now?' she asked, cradling his jaw in her hand, and he smiled.

It was a bit crooked, but it was there. 'I think so. It's still a work in progress, but I'm getting there.' He turned his head and kissed her hand, then stood up. 'I need to go and finish off in the kitchen.'

'Want any help?'

'No, you stay here and talk to the dogs. I won't be long.'

He warmed the food up, stirring it gently on the hob, blanched the green beans, drained the baby new potatoes and laid the table.

Nothing fancy, no candles, since it was four in the afternoon and candles might look a bit ridiculous. And he checked his back pocket, just in case.

Lord, he was nervous. What if—

'Are you sure I can't help?'

He turned and smiled, or tried to, but it was probably a pretty poor effort. 'No, you're fine, I'm done. Come and sit down.'

She sat, watching him curiously. 'Smells good,' she said, and he put the dishes down on the table and took the lid off the casserole dish.

She looked at it, then up at him, her heart starting to race.

'Is that…what I think it is?'

She saw his throat work as he swallowed. 'Yes, it is.'

He'd cooked her Marry Me Chicken?

She looked away, wondering if…then looked back up at him. Was she imagining it, or did he look nervous? She'd *never* seen Hugo look nervous. And now he was fumbling in his back pocket, pulling something out.

A—ring?

He knelt down beside her and met her eyes, and she bit her lips and tried not to cry.

'I love you, Eleanor Radcliffe,' he said, his voice low, soft and a little shaky. 'I know I'm a basket case, but I'm working on it, and I promise you that whatever happens, whatever goes wrong, whatever life throws at us, I will *always* love you. Will you marry me?'

'What about children?' she asked, not because she wanted them, but because she needed to hear his answer, whatever it was, before she gave him hers.

'What about them? If you want my children, then if it happens, I'm fine with it. More than fine. Yes, it might hurt, but it would also heal, and I'd love us to be a family. But there's no hurry, and I don't mind either way, so long as I've got you. But the thought of you with another man…' He hauled in a breath. 'I wouldn't try to stop you if it was what you wanted, but it would break my heart if I knew I'd driven you into someone else's arms.'

She cradled his cheek in her hand. 'I can't give you Samuel back, you do know that, don't you?' she said gently, unable even to imagine the depth of his pain, but he just smiled a sad little smile.

'Of course I do, and I wouldn't want that. He

was incredibly special to me, but we always knew we would lose him. What I didn't know was how much it was possible to love someone so small, and how much it would hurt to lose them.'

'Oh, Hugo…'

'Don't be sad for me. I'm OK. And if you want to have a family, we can do that, but I don't want to put any pressure on you one way or the other. I just need to be with you. That's all I ask. Anything else would be a bonus.'

She leant in and kissed him, just a gentle touch, then sat back.

'I was coming back to tell you that I don't need to have a baby to make me happy. Yes, I'd always hoped that one day I'd meet a man, the sort of man who wouldn't leave me like my father left my mother, and that we'd get married and have a family, but nobody's ever made me feel even remotely like this before. I fell in love with you weeks ago, and then I found out you'd lost a baby, and my heart just broke for you.'

'Oh, Ellie…'

'I can't replace him for you, I know that, and I know you'll always feel a tinge of sadness around babies, but, children or no children, I want to be with you. I love you, Hugo. I know it's ridiculously quick, but I think I've loved you since you saved Lola's life and we sat and had that long talk and I realised what a truly decent and wonderful human being you are.'

He gave a choked laugh. 'Don't go too mad, I'm very far from perfect.'

She smiled at him, the love of her life. 'Aren't we all? I still love you. And yes, I'll marry you, of course I will. I'd be honoured.'

'I thought you'd never get round to saying that,' he said, and he started to laugh, then his eyes softened and he took her hand.

'I don't know if this will fit you. It—' He broke off and swallowed hard. 'It was my mother's engagement ring, and I know she'd be so happy for you to wear it. She would have loved you very much, and so would my father.'

'Even though I'm a vet?'

He smiled. 'Even though you're a vet.'

He slid the ring onto her finger, and it fitted as if it had been made for her. She looked down at it, a row of five simple but beautifully cut graduated diamonds, sparkling in the light. She touched it with shaking fingers, and bit her lip to try and stop the tears.

'It's beautiful,' she said. 'Thank you.'

He stood up and pulled her to her feet, and he wrapped her in his arms and held her as if he'd never let her go.

'Make love to me, Hugo,' she said, and the meaning wasn't lost on him.

'Nothing would make me happier.'

He put the lid back on the casserole dish with a smile. There'd be time to eat it later, but right now they had better things to do, and its job was done…

EPILOGUE

ANOTHER SCORCHING EARLY September day, just like it had been this time last year for their wedding day.

Hugo locked the gates and the front door, ran upstairs and showered, pulled on shorts and a T-shirt and went out into the garden.

A year ago, there'd been a marquee on the lawn for their wedding reception. They'd closed the practice at lunchtime on that Friday so all the staff could join them, and he and Ellie had had a quiet wedding with all the people that mattered to them.

Peter and Sally, of course, and Ellie's mother and her partner from Spain; Jim Harkness, all the practice staff, old friends—nobody had been left out. Ellie wore his mother's ring, he his father's dress watch, and in his breast pocket against his heart he had a picture of Samuel—they'd all been there in their thoughts and in their hearts.

And since then, there'd been a new arrival.

He could see them in the shade under the copper beech. Ellie had spread a rug on the grass, and they were all lying on it, Ellie on her side, head propped up on one hand, watching Lola and Rufus, who were, in turn, lying with their heads on their front paws and watching the newest member of the family.

She'd been born so fast he'd delivered her himself on the bathroom floor, bright red and screaming with rage and utterly beautiful. It was a moment he'd been dreading, but it had been the best and most wonderful moment of his life.

The dogs lifted their heads and wagged their tails as he walked barefoot across the grass towards them, and he stopped and looked down at them all with a wry smile, his heart filled with love.

'You all look very relaxed,' he said, and knelt down beside Ellie and gave her a kiss. 'Everything OK?'

'Very OK, thank you. It's blissful.'

'How long's she been asleep?'

'I'm not sure. I fed her a little while ago but I'm sure she wouldn't say no to a cuddle.'

He smiled. 'I can't wake her, she needs her sleep and so do I. She was up most of the night.'

'Tell me about it.' She shuffled across and made room for him, and he lay down between them and drew her into his arms and kissed her.

'I love you, Mrs Alexander.'

'I love you, too. I'm glad it's the weekend, we've missed you.'

'I was never far away.' He kissed her again, his body stirring, but he ignored it. It wasn't the only thing stirring, and he snagged another kiss and propped himself up so he could look down at their baby. Charlotte, after his mother, but Lottie to them.

'Hello, my gorgeous girl,' he crooned softly, and she kicked her legs and smiled at him, just the way Samuel used to.

He swallowed the lump in his throat, scooped her up and cradled her in the crook of his arm. She was so precious, so easy to love, but it hadn't been easy. The first few weeks of the pregnancy he'd lived on a knife-edge, and only after the first scan had he dared to believe in her. And here she was, perfect in every way, three months old and the image of her mother, and he loved her more than he would ever have believed possible.

'Now, little Lottie, listen to your daddy,' he murmured, still smiling. 'You need to be a good girl tonight and sleep, because it's our wedding anniversary and we would like to celebrate it by sleeping all night…'

'*All* night?'

He dragged his eyes off the baby and looked at Ellie—his wife, his soulmate, his saviour. And he smiled.

'Well, maybe not *all* night…'

* * * * *

If you enjoyed this story, check out these other great reads from Caroline Anderson

Finding Their Forever Family
The Midwife's Miracle Twins
Healing Her Emergency Doc
Tempted by the Single Mom

All available now!

HARLEQUIN
Reader Service

Enjoyed your book?

Try the perfect subscription for Romance readers and get more great books like this delivered right to your door.

See why over 10+ million readers have tried Harlequin Reader Service.

Start with a Free Welcome Collection with free books and a gift—valued over $20.

Choose any series in print or ebook.
See website for details and order today:

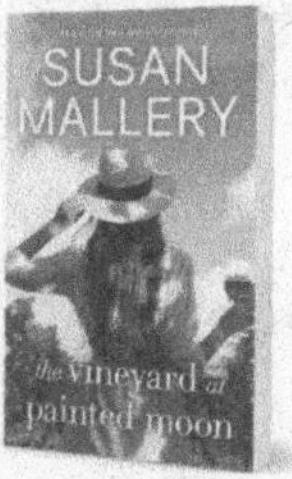

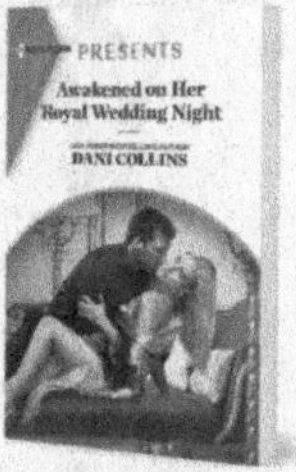

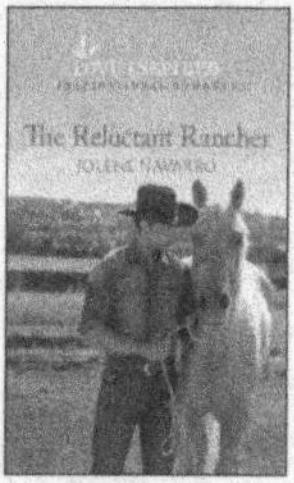

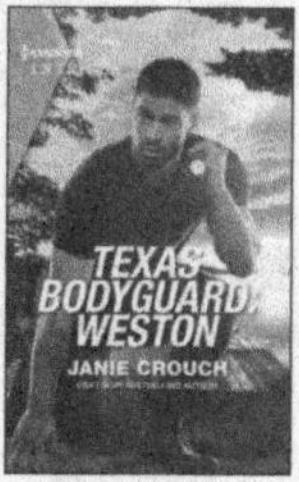

TryReaderService.com/subscriptions

RSBPA24R